YOUNG
@ ANY AGE

SECRETS TO SLOWING THE AGING PROCESS

WILL LOISEAU

Copyright © 2024 by WL Media

All rights reserved. No part of this book may be reproduced or used in any manner without the prior written permission of the copyright owner, except for the use of brief quotations in a book review.

Editor *Carol Edwards*

Cover Designer *Shannen Craft*

Graphic Design *Kristen Rinner*

Book Interior Designer *Shah Nawaz*

Photographs *courtesy of the author's achieves, Jonathan Mok, and Madison Fender*

DEDICATION

Dedicated to my amazing parents, Wilfrid and Alberte, whose youthful spirits inspired this work. With eternal gratitude for the priceless gift of your wisdom and love.

CONTENTS

A Message to the Reader — 1

Introduction — 2

Why I Wrote This Book — 4

1. Bronchitis in Brooklyn: Navigating the Fog of Illness — 8

2. Haitian Household: Family, Food, and Roots — 11

3. Rediscover Nature: Seeds of Wisdom, Blooms of Experience — 20

4. Sign of the Times: Freshman Fast Food Chronicles — 26

5. Preventable Dis-ease: Questioning Conventional Health Wisdom — 32

6. Catching a Cold: Unlearning and Relearning Health — 45

7. The Illusion of Labels: The Hidden Realities Behind Titles — 53

8. Self-Medication: Maneuvering Life in a Haze of Intoxication — 59

9. Change: The Email That Altered My Path — 69

10. Fast or Slow: Hitting Life's Reset Button — 76

11. Toothache to Triumph: Healing from Within, One Bite at a Time — 85

12. Redemption in Red: A Battle Against Eye Agony — 94

13. Embracing the Power of Self-Discovery — 103

14. Solar Symphony: Dancing with the Energy of Life — 115

15. Youth Rediscovered: Balancing Responsibilities and Dreams — 121

16. Black Don't Crack: Decoding the Myths and Realities of Ageless Beauty — 124

17. Year of the Return: A Homecoming Celebration	140
18. Sole Searching: Discovering Ability Where I Least Expected	150
19. The Miseducation of Will Loiseau	162
20. Salty Secrets: Lessons on Sodium and Health	173
21. Shopping Carts Full of Symptoms: Hidden in Plain Sight	185
22. Aging Gracefully: Embracing the Tapestry of Life's Journey	199
23. Down to Earth: My Earthing Exploration	206
24. Final Thoughts	210
Sources	216
Exercises To Improve Posture	218
Recipes	220
Simple Quiz Questions	227
Acknowledgements	229
About The Author	231

A MESSAGE TO THE READER

Dear Reader,

It is my sincere hope that you may find this book enriching. Within these pages, I share opinions, ideas, and suggestions in a spirit of helpfulness. If anything, herein brings you joy or positively impacts your life, it would bring me joy as well.

However, I am not a licensed professional, and this book is not meant to replace individualized guidance from your doctor or other qualified advisor. They know your unique needs best. Before making significant lifestyle changes, I encourage you to consult them.

Great care has gone into researching and writing this book, but there is always a chance of unintentional errors or oversights. Please apply your own good judgment when considering the contents. This is my story and these are my results. I cannot control how this advice is interpreted or implemented, so no guarantees are given regarding your results. I don't assume liability for choices made after reading this book.

Your health and wellbeing depend most on the partnership between you and your chosen experts. I hope this book provides value as you make positive changes, but please reach out to professionals whenever needed. Their guidance is essential as you determine what is right for you.

My goal is to share these ideas respectfully, with your wellbeing in mind. I wish you all the best on your journey.

Best of health,
Will Loiseau

INTRODUCTION

Life is like a shadow and a mist; it passes quickly by, and is no more.
— *African proverb*

Death is not a curse. We will die. No pill, potion, diet plan, or book written by yours truly will change that. In the meantime, we should live as happily as possible. Health is the center of gravity of happiness for everyone. Therefore, the "pursuit of happiness" should be the pursuit of health. Breaking the world record for the longest-lived person may not be on our wish lists. But what if we could increase life span while extending health span, the period in our lives when we are most active?

Slowing down the aging process begins with the will to live. Cherishing this life and learning as much as possible from our experiences is essential. Finding our purpose opens unlimited possibilities to thrive. There lies the reason to endure. Trillions of cells have come together to create us. They are programmed to self-preserve. Unlike other animals, we have freedom to choose from a variety of options. Certain choices allow some of us to age gracefully and remain healthy into our golden years, while other courses of action influence struggle with chronic pain and rapid cognitive decline. Throughout these pages I will share events that have led me to conclude that we can become healthier with each passing year. I've had the pleasure to learn from and consult with people from all walks of life around the world. We are all unique but share much more in common.

Don't underestimate yourself. Within us all lies the potential for a healthier life. Living outside of the comfort zone of poor lifestyle choices can produce life-changing results moving forward.

Eat healthy. Get exercise. Drink water. Sound familiar? We live in a world where information is easily accessible. What was it about this book that piqued your interest? Are you or someone you know in need of inspiration? Maybe you want confirmation that your lifestyle is whole. There are levels toward the pinnacle. Optimum overall health development requires consistent practice, and get this: There's no chance of perfection. That's right. We're all part of an imperfect planet. Our rapidly changing environment is a direct reflection of the choices our species has made, for the better and the worst. We have the ability to manifest greatness. Let's strive happily for our wellness and betterment.

WHY I WROTE THIS BOOK

There's a God force inside of you that gives you a will to live.
— *Dick Gregory*

In grade school I was taught that Juan Ponce de León, a Spanish explorer, sailed to Florida in 1513, searching for the Fountain of Youth. I was captivated by the concept. I'd been to the fountains at malls and museums where people threw loose change in the water. For some, seeing their coin next to other coins is a way to socially connect with people they've never met. Others believe that if they make a wish, the water's memory will make it come true. Was there an actual fountain that could suspend time and keep us all younger? I wondered. *The Fountain of Youth* is also the name of an oil painting by German artist Lucas Cranach. In it he pictures women bathing in a fountain during the Middle Ages. Older women are bathing on one side of the fountain. As they move from one side to the other, they appear more youthful and rejuvenated. If there really were such a thing, I wanted to find it and bathe in it. Subconsciously, I've been on a quest to find the best ways to preserve youth.

I've lost count of how many times I've been mistaken for being years younger than my actual age. It's happened all over the world—in different states, countries, and even continents. People are always surprised when I reveal my birth date. At first, I thought it was just good genes. Let's be clear: They do play a role. But as it happened more and more frequently, I began to wonder if there was something more to it. Was the universe trying to send me a message?

For years, I tried to fit in with societal norms. I followed the latest trends, ate what everyone else was eating, and bought into the promises of the health and fitness industry. But despite my best efforts, I still suffered from all the common ailments of modern society. It wasn't until I started listening to my inner voice that things began to change.

You see, I believe that we all possess innate wisdom—a voice that knows what's best for us, if only we're willing to listen. Listening to that inner voice became my compass, guiding me toward a different approach to aging and health. It wasn't about conforming to external standards or following the latest trends. It was about tapping into my own unique needs and finding what truly worked for me. And the more I listened, the easier it became to discover the secrets to youth at any age.

We start aging from the time we're born. As we grow older, we tend to value our health more. Those of us fortunate to have them remember the day we spotted that first gray hair looking back at us in the mirror. As the years pass, we notice the things we are no longer able to do as easily. Many of us are losing our health earlier than people in preceding generations. Sadly, it is no longer uncommon for parents to outlive their offspring.

My firsthand experiences before, during, and after the devastating 2010 earthquake in Port-au-Prince, Haiti, instilled in me a sense of urgency to uncover solutions that could benefit everyone. I was driven to find answers to why so many individuals around me were struggling with compromised health. While natural disasters are beyond our control, I noticed something intriguing upon returning to the United States. It became apparent that I had more opportunities to improve and maintain my personal health than I had previously realized. Despite searching far and wide, I could not find a book that offered what you are reading right now. I decided to take it upon myself to fill that gap. After all, what is the use of great health if those we love are not around to enjoy it with us? Undoubtedly, good health is true wealth. This book is not a panacea that can solve everyone's problems. No single effort can achieve that. However, my story will resonate with those who are eager to see, experience, and make a difference in their lives.

Throughout this book, I have sprinkled what I call "GEMS." These are actions that anyone can immediately implement in their daily routines. GEMS have made healthier living much easier for me to maintain. They have provided me with gradual effective measurable solutions (GEMS) that have changed my life for the better.

If you're looking for a quick fix to solve chronic health problems or slow down aging, this book may not help you. I've been asked on many occasions to summarize the key to health in one sentence. While the concept is simple, it hasn't been so easy for me to explain. That's why I decided to elaborate on this canvas.

Having said that, writing is the best way for me to detail my personal choices to promote health and combat disease. In search of answers, I began a quest for knowledge so others would not have to experience the pain of losing family members, friends, and loved ones prematurely. This book is for those who feel powerless against poor health. Good health cannot be outsourced to a personal trainer, nutritionist, health guru, or a medical doctor. It won't ever fit in a capsule.

Why do I believe that I'm qualified to speak on aging? As someone who has experienced and successfully overcome the typical age-related symptoms, spent years working in the health-care and wellness industry, volunteered in hospitals, consulted with doctors, nutritionists, and chiropractors, and worked in assisted-living facilities, I have amassed a wealth of knowledge on how to maintain youthfulness and vitality as we age. In addition, as a certified personal trainer and holistic sports nutrition consultant, I have helped numerous individuals attain their health objectives. Based on my extensive background, I'm confident in my ability to share effective solutions that have helped me overcome the common issues that accompany aging.

1

BRONCHITIS IN BROOKLYN: NAVIGATING THE FOG OF ILLNESS

The first breath is the beginning of death.
— *Anonymous*

The view was breathtaking. My sleepy eyes squinted up at bright halogen streetlights. Blurry wide rays of orange light beamed down on me. I was lying on my back in the rear seat, or maybe it was a black hole, or it could've been a web spun by a funnel-web spider. Gasping for air, I closed my eyes and held on for as long as I could. The previous cough stunned me like a right uppercut from Iron Mike in the first round. My body was getting battered by the storm.

"Aaah" was the sound I emitted, gritting my teeth as I inhaled against my will. I grabbed the seat and braced myself. "Chooo!" followed as I violently exhaled.

It hurt to sneeze through my irritated throat. But no matter how hard I tried, I couldn't hold them in. I could hear my heart thumping in stereo. It doubled the rhythm of the rapid-moving windshield wipers. At the stoplight, autumn precipitation tap-danced on the car's exterior. Red break lights and steamy headlights reflected off of the fog. Church Avenue was desolate. Everything around me seemed like a dreadful dream. My father didn't say much. Although he seemed calm, I felt his nervous energy as he gripped the wheel. With a noble sense of purpose, he navigated through the slick, rainy streets of Kings County, New York.

"We're almost there. Can you sit up?" my mom asked with stern concern.

"I'm trying," I mumbled, peeling myself off of the seat.

Every minute she kept asking questions I could barely respond to. This was the feeling of being at the mercy of dis-ease. Each inhale was of limited capacity, constricted by something that wouldn't allow me to draw breath without a wheeze. Imagine having someone control your lungs, limiting how deeply you could breathe. I was physically drained. If this was what growing pains felt like, I was curious how long this would last. As powerful as this force was, it didn't stop me from believing that we'd make it to the hospital. Brookdale was blocks away from where we lived on East Ninety-second Street.

It was after 3:00 A.M. Waiting in the emergency room for what felt like time without end, my parents' facial expressions spelled exhaustion. In a few hours, one of them would have to go to work. I felt guilty for interrupting their sleep. But tonight, I was feeling the wrath of another attack of asthmatic bronchitis.

I'd never seen either of my parents smoke or suffer from anything like this. Even though they both were always there for me, I felt cold and alone. Pain is inevitable on the journey of life. But only I knew what it felt like in my body. I stepped on a stool and sat up on the paper-covered exam table. Every time the doctor placed the stethoscope on my chest and back, it was icy. I'd flinch whenever it first made contact with the goose bumps on my skin. A few minutes later, there was a prescription paper waiting for us to pick up at the front desk. I couldn't figure out why the handwritten scribble on the paper was so hard to read. Maybe the doctor was a graffiti writer in his off-hours. The paper had the name and address of the nearest pharmacy and special instructions from the doctor. It included details on how much and how frequently to take what was in the vial of pills with chemical ingredients. The sum of these ingredients was supposed to make me feel better.

Vivid recollections like these remind me of some of the formidable challenges I faced early in my life. At the tender age of seven, I found myself burdened with a weariness that surpassed my years, as if my lungs had aged prematurely. Questions swirled around in my young mind: Why was this happening? Would mucus and medication become a way of life for me? Little did I know then that the topic of health and its intricate relationship with aging would become an inseparable part of my journey. These memories, etched deep within the fabric of my being, serve as indelible markers, signifying the beginning of personal narratives that will gradually unravel the intricate tapestry of my existence. My purpose in sharing the following stories of self-discovery, resilience, and triumphant defiance over adversity is to inspire and empower others. Within each of us lies a wellspring of transformative powers waiting to be discovered.

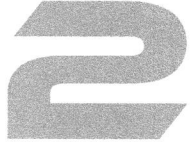

HAITIAN HOUSEHOLD: FAMILY, FOOD, AND ROOTS

Sa ou fè, se li ou wè (What you do is what you see.)
— Haitian proverb

Around the time when "8th Wonder," by the Sugarhill Gang, first graced the mainstream radio waves, my parents and I were visiting family in New Jersey. My older cousin Anderson, who was almost two years older than I was, pulled out a vinyl record from its paper sleeve in the living room cabinet. The record had a baby blue circle sticker in the middle, adorned with a colorful design that immediately caught my attention.

"Have you heard this yet?" Anderson asked me with a confident grin as he placed the record on the turntable.

"No. What is it?" I inquired, curious to know.

"This song is everything right now," he replied, lowering the stylus onto the record grooves.

Excitement filled the room as a vibrant voice leaped off the vinyl, commanding us to surrender to the infectious rhythm of the track, igniting an irresistible urge within us all to clap our hands in unison. This was my introduction to a genre called Hip Hop. But our moms, calling from the dining room, interrupted our musical escapade.

"Anderson! Wilfrid! *Vini manje.*" Come and eat.

Whenever we gathered around the dinner table, it was always a joyous occasion. Sharing food was a cherished ritual for us. Our place mats were adorned with colorful pictures of fruits, adding a vibrant touch to the otherwise brown-and-beige-dominated plates. Uncle Ben's brown rice, kidney beans, boiled or fried plantains, along with chicken, beef, or griot—a Haitian delicacy— were the staple dishes. A small dish of iceberg lettuce and tomato salad sat on the side of the table, looking somewhat lonely. And next to it was a bowl filled with plastic apple, banana, and grape ornaments, adding a playful touch to our mealtime ambience.

I wasn't a fan of griot and would try to hide it whenever it was served. As the adults encouraged us to eat our salads first, I would pick at the meat with my knife and fork, waiting for the perfect opportunity to sneak it off my plate. Anderson, on the other hand, loved griot and would ask for any that I didn't want. Even with the added gravy, I couldn't stand the stringy, chewy texture in my mouth. Despite my dislike for the dish, the love and warmth of the shared meal made it all worth it.

Years later, I grew more adventurous in trying new foods that the rest of the family enjoyed, including various meats, like poultry, beef, and pork. However, my body always had the strongest negative reactions to seafood. One night, after trying a small piece of fish at the dinner table, my tongue and face began to swell, and my airways felt like they were closing in. I gasped for air, and my parents rushed me to the nearest hospital. After that traumatic experience, the mere smell of fish at the market made me feel sick.

Just the sight of a dead fish staring back at me with its lifeless eyes sent shivers down my spine.

I couldn't help but wonder if the diseases responsible for afflicting my loved ones and me were somehow lurking in fish. That must have been why my body reacted so severely. Whenever headlines claiming to fight these diseases flashed across the television screen, I couldn't help but pay attention.

"Mom, come see this!" I'd call from the living room.

"What is it?" she'd reply, running from the kitchen.

"There's a new thing they said can cure diabetes."

"Oh yeah. What's the name?"

"The newsman on channel two just said it. Something about F . . . D . . . A? They'll give the name after the commercials. Maybe you can get some at your hospital."

"Call me when it starts." she said, returning to check on the chicken cooking in the oven.

My mother was a registered nurse at Long Island College Hospital in Brooklyn. That was where I was born. I figured she'd be in the best position to find a cure for her disease. She was at the hospital a lot. That place was filled with doctors and other nurses. They were the specialists who always had those new gadgets that were supposed to cure people. For some reason, they didn't always work.

If disease was responsible for making people look and feel older, something had to be done about it. My curious nature had me searching for clues way before I understood what I was searching for. I began to notice a few things after we finished dinner. My mother would take the corn oil from the pan she had fried chicken in and pour it into a large glass jar. Sometimes, she would use an empty plastic corn oil container. The oil became darker after cooking and was peppered with black sediment. Once the oil cooled down, a thick layer of tan-colored fat would form on the surface of the oil. It grossed me out. I asked her why she did it. She told me the oil was still good to reuse. It was also a way to save money. I didn't get it. When I visited my friends, I paid closer attention to what their parents did. Maybe it was a Black or Caribbean custom, because Marcel, Jean, and Sandra's mothers all did it, too. It was a strange practice, but I saw it being done so frequently in my surroundings, I got used to it.

After finishing a plate of fried plantains, I would head to the kitchen to place my plate in the sink. However, I would often get scolded by my dad for not first wiping the oil off the plate with a paper towel. He would stress how the oil could congeal and clog the pipes if poured down the drain. I didn't understand why it was a problem, since we consumed the same oil in our food. It didn't make sense to me at the time. Little did I know that the damage caused by the accumulation of oil in the pipes was a potential indicator of the harm it could cause to our bodies. A person's lymphatic system, much like the plumbing in our homes, could also become clogged, leading to potential health emergencies.

As I grew older, I realized that our parents had always acted with good intentions when it came to our health. They fed us the best way they knew how, based on what they had been taught when they were younger. I didn't hold any resentment toward them. In fact, I became increasingly intrigued by our health habits, or sometimes lack thereof, and developed a strong desire to learn more about how to adopt a healthier lifestyle.

Childhood was a time of exploration with unrefined, animal instincts. My developing brain was a cerebral sponge, soaking up everything my senses could absorb. I didn't fully understand the relationship between living animals and what was presented to me whenever it was time to eat. I had one foot in a world where food wasn't a priority when my friends and I played outdoors. The other foot was in the rich culture I was being taught by my loving family. For them, food was of utmost importance. The dinner table was where stories were told, problems were discussed, and future habits were formed. Food was how we got together and strengthened as a unit. As we grew, we continued to be shaped by our surroundings.

On the first day of each year, our families and close friends would come together to eat soup. I loved hearing stories from my father about our history. Food was always a part of those stories. He would tell me how important it was to understand where we came from, to understand who we were. He read many books on world history.

"Why do we always eat the same soup on New Year's?" I asked him.

"The French used to control Saint-Domingue. This is pumpkin soup. Haitians were treated less than dogs. The white slave owners would throw the food they didn't want at them on the floor."

"How long did this happen?"

"Many years. Haiti went to war."

"Against the French?"

"Of course. The French, the British, and the Spanish, too."

"We beat them all?"

"Yes. In 1804, Jean-Jacques Dessalines led the army. He beat the French. He changed the name of the island to Ayiti. It means 'many mountains.' The first Black nation in the world to win independence."

"All by themselves?"

"Yes. They were the first in the world to say no more slavery."

"So, why do we eat this soup?"

"They never let Haitians eat the soup. But we were the people who made the soup. They treated us like we were nothing. Now we eat soup every year. Soup joumou means independence."

As I got older, I started to see the connections between food, culture, and history. I saw how the things we ate and the way we prepared them were linked to our past. Before long, I also began to crave the same foods everyone around me ate. My palate became conditioned to eating more fried foods, animal foods, and refined carbohydrates.

My family held those in certain professions in high regard, including lawyers, engineers, and especially doctors and nurses. These careers were viewed as stable, well paying, and respectable, and were the main paths of choice for Haitian immigrants who arrived in the United States and Canada during the 1960s. A few times a year, my mother, father, and I would fall ill with something, whether it was the flu, a cold, fever, or some other minor ailment. As my mother was a medical professional, I trusted her ability to handle our health crises. However, it seemed odd that my mother was diagnosed with type 2 diabetes mellitus when she was in her forties. The doctors explained that her pancreas was producing enough insulin, but her body was unable to properly use the sugar in her bloodstream, leading to a range of symptoms and complications over time. They never investigated what could be preventing the sugar from entering the cells or asked about her lifestyle choices outside of the hospital. Although my mother worked long hours, that wasn't all she did. They never once inquired about what she ate. Instead, they attributed her condition to genetics and told her that diabetes was an inevitable life sentence that required a lifetime of synthetic insulin and other medications.

My mother's coworkers, who were mostly Haitian nurses, also had chronic health issues. They seemed to wear their diagnoses with a sense of pride, having been formally taught in nursing school how to manage their symptoms and medications. However, there was no emphasis on the role of lifestyle in managing their disease symptoms, and this omission continued throughout their education. Coming from religious households, they believed that their faith would always see them through any difficulties. It was rare for them to be diagnosed with chronic disease before migrating to the United States. The nurses were often years younger than the patients they treated, as type 2 diabetes, arthritis, cancer, and hypertension were considered older person's diseases during the 1980s and 1990s. At that time, they were not as prevalent in American society or globally as they are today.

In Haiti, people relied on *doktè fèy*, or leaf doctors, to treat common illnesses with natural remedies derived from plants. They recognized the unique properties and benefits those plants offered for healing. However, as Haitians migrated to the United States and Canada, they became increasingly disconnected from their natural roots. The medical education and career paths they pursued took them further away from plant-based medicine. What they didn't realize was that the cost of their success was high. As medical professionals, they ended up prescribing and taking the same synthetic chemicals they administered to their patients. They may have been taking different dosage amounts and they may not have been officially diagnosed. They may have still been able to enjoy the freedom of working on their feet, but they were slowly losing touch with their roots in the process.

As a child, I noticed that many of the nurses in the hospital were overweight. I wondered if this was a result of their lifestyle in the United States or if it was something else. However, I didn't know how to ask without offending them. I observed silently, trying to understand the profession's demands. From what I could tell, nursing required physical and mental strength. Nurses worked long, demanding twelve-hour shifts, with limited breaks. They had to organize piles of paperwork, walk quickly, practice patience and empathy, and pay attention to detail at all times.

In Haiti, there was no mass production of farm animals. My father would often tell me about how he fed the animals he grew up with leftover food scraps. There were no genetically modified crops, synthetic hormones, antibiotic injections, or cramped cages. When my parents arrived in the United States during the civil rights movement, the food industry was beginning to promote convenience. My parents were astounded by the size of the chickens on grocery store shelves. These chickens were twice as big as anything they had ever seen before. They were also taken aback by jumbo-size eggs, which they had never encountered before. As new citizens, their tax dollars were subsidizing these products. Their relationship with food began to shift in their new surroundings. What was once an occasional delicacy had become cheap and abundant enough to eat multiple times a day. Consequently, they developed conflicting identities with regard to food and lifestyle. In Haiti, walking miles every day in warm, tropical weather and eating off the land was the norm, and everyone was thin.

However, in the big city, driving and public transportation became popular options, and the definition of "good" eating became distorted. Haitians began adapting to comfort foods and American capitalism, and increased body fat became a sign of improved finances and food abundance at home. This was especially true for Haitian women, who had higher rates of diabetes. If someone was perceived as too slim, they were less attractive to Haitian men and could be mistaken for a "zombie," a sickly thin person. Jokes within the community would poke fun at slim physiques, with critiques like *"Vant ou ap touche do ou,"* meaning "Your stomach is touching your back." But as soon as someone became noticeably overweight, they would hear *"Bouch ou plen. Ou pa ka kanpe,"* meaning "Your mouth is full of food. You can't even stand up." While these comments may have been meant as lighthearted humor, they held some truth and confusion beneath the surface. The emphasis on physical movement and caloric moderation had shifted, and culture shock was occurring in real time.

GEMS: The more I learn about Haitian history, the more awe and reverence I feel for my ancestral lineage. Their courage, strength, and ingenuity in the face of oppression leave me humbled. I've gradually made changes to the dishes from my childhood - like soup joumou - by using healthier ingredients. My goal isn't to drastically alter the recipes, but to celebrate the essence of the cuisine through a conscious lifestyle. This allows me to celebrate the culture while adhering to my evolving nutritional needs.

Rice and I have a long-distance relationship these days. Depending on how it's cultivated, rice has been known to contain arsenic, lead, and other heavy metals. High blood pressure, skin diseases, and neurological issues have all been linked to long-term consumption of heavy metals. Besides, I can no longer tolerate the food-induced coma feeling or "itis" I get every time I finish eating large amounts of starchy grains. I no longer prioritize anything that drains my energy. I've since learned to either prepare quinoa or bloom wild rice. These substitutes are easy to make and are much healthier alternatives. Check the recipe section at the end of this book for more details.

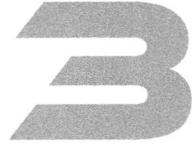

REDISCOVER NATURE: SEEDS OF WISDOM, BLOOMS OF EXPERIENCE

Love the world as your own self; then you can truly care for all things.
— *Lao Tzu*

The crack epidemic swept through Brooklyn and the rest of New York City like a wild tornado. Desperate fiends broke into our apartment twice in less than two years, and violent crime was on the rise. It became dangerous for me even to play with my toys on the front porch. My parents decided that they had had enough and relocated us farther east. As an adolescent growing up on Long Island, my new friends and I would practically live outdoors. The warmer the temperatures got after the brutally cold winters, the more we would wander into unknown territories. One of our favorite pastimes was riding our BMX (bicycle motocross) bikes around town and into the woods. Bay Shore was where folks from NYC would go to get away from all the frantic energy. Members of the working class began their home-ownership journeys, while the wealthy would purchase second homes and investment properties. This was a way to access the beaches on the north and south shores easily.

During the 1980s and 1990s, there were acres and acres of undeveloped land, especially the farther we went into eastern Suffolk County. The trees became our close family members. We would enjoy the fresh scents of evergreens and the protection the white oak trees provided from heavy rains. We even climbed red maple trees to relax and get a bird's-eye view of our surroundings. Little did I know there was just as much life teeming right under our feet. The trees interacted with their neighbors through mycelium, an extensive underground network of fungi. The trees did so much more than add beauty to our landscape. They were a part of our extended community. They protected one another from disease and other threats by exchanging nutrients while we were at play above the surface. I interacted with my friends with verbal and nonverbal language. The trees communicated with one another by releasing pheromones, plant chemicals that also affected us in beneficial ways. We felt better whenever we were outside, breathing oxygen from the trees. I guess they were relaying information to us, too. I often wondered how old they were. Some of the tall ones must have experienced hundreds of seasons. Being at one with nature was the ultimate high. We would mount our BMX bikes, jump ramps, perform freestyle tricks, and go on adventures to find new trails in the woods. I always wondered when and how these trails were created. Were they forged by prehistoric dinosaurs, or was it by the deer we'd see scatter away from time to time? Some trails were wide; others were narrow. Some were filled with dirt and rocks, others were layered with autumn leaves, and a few would lead to dead ends.

We didn't care if it was windy, raining, or snowing. The sounds of rustling leaves and sticks snapping under our thin tires as we sped through the forest were awesome. The trails would serve as shortcuts to cross town, travel to a friend's house, or hide out and find our identities in nature. When differences had to be settled, the great outdoors even served as a fighting ring.

Losing our direction, getting spooked out by weird sounds, unfamiliar wildlife, and feeling the nervousness of the unknown formed a major part of our childhoods. It worked out for the better that our parents didn't know all of the trouble we got into. Adventures through exploration were what allowed us to build confidence, develop our senses, and learn outside of the classroom. That's how we learned to read the clouds, listen for thunder, and gauge when and where a rainstorm was headed. Trying to remember which trail led back home before the sun went down was exciting, especially when the nervous pit in my stomach helped me to navigate heavily wooded, unbeaten paths. These activities served to sharpen my memory and attention to detail. My companions and I had to use parts of the brain we normally didn't use to make decisions, acting instinctively instead.

Gardening was one of my father's favorite hobbies. Around the time I started high school, he'd spontaneously make me drop whatever I was doing to help him gather tools. We'd get shovels, gloves, hoes, hand rakes, trowels, and hit the dirt. He taught me how to plant strawberries, cucumbers, tomatoes, lettuce, zucchini, and peppers in the small backyard garden. At first, I thought gardening was boring. I couldn't find the instantaneous action and excitement that bike riding gave me. But then I picked up on a few things that seemed to encourage the plants to grow faster and be healthier. Soil preparation, distance between plants, water requirements for each variety of plant, the role of worms and other organisms, sunlight preferences, and patience were all important. The more involved I was with the process, the more I understood the attention to detail required to assist nature in its expression. Time seemed to move at a different speed whenever we interacted with nature. The pace seemed somewhat slower. But that reduction in speed was necessary for me to appreciate my surroundings. Being outside invited us to breathe more deeply than we typically did indoors. There were few distractions and so much to pay attention to. The birds, rabbits, squirrels, frogs, snakes, and other animals were all attentive to what we were doing. Television and video games were predictable and scripted, but out in nature no two days were exactly alike. Watching the plants grow at their steady tempo was gratifying. We literally enjoyed the fruits of our labor. Zucchini and lettuce may not have been my favorites, but I noticed a difference between what we grew and what we bought at the store. The store-bought vegetables were bigger, but what we grew was fresher and tasted better. The more we ate from the garden, the more we fine-tuned our abilities to discern different flavors and textures. Identifying these characteristics is one of the skills we cultivated when we were younger. No two fruits were identical in taste, even if they were the same variety. Each fruit had its own unique character. This is also true of humans, of course.

A few friends of mine, who resided on the same block but did not attend my school, had an obsession with science. They were nerds in their own universe. While my classmates were into the latest clothes, sneakers, and music, these kids stayed dirty while digging in the dirt or searching for anything that moved in the mud. At first, I thought they were strange, but their passion to explore was contagious. It wasn't long before I'd occasionally start changing my clothes after school and getting my fingernails in the earth, too. The life science I learned outside of the classroom was so much more fun. Our imaginations had no boundaries. We educated ourselves about the small creatures around us and their roles in nature. By using action figures and role playing, we incorporated nature into our microworld. I didn't like houseflies buzzing near my ears or hovering over my food, but they were a necessity. They broke down organic matter. So did the fungi under our feet in the forest. The larvae of fireflies eat slugs and worms to help balance our ecosystem. We call fireflies "lightning bugs" because of the cool yellow light they emit from their abdomens. Catching a dozen or so in glass jars and watching them scintillate at night were our versions of lanterns. Crickets chirped so loudly at night. Whenever I tried to tiptoe closer and pinpoint their location, they'd get silent. Crickets help to keep the wasp populations in check and improve the soil quality. Cicadas were loud, too. They prune trees and provide fertilizer to the rest of the forest when they die. Once in a while I'd spot a praying mantis. They eat roaches and mosquitoes. Ladybugs were good for keeping pests off the green lettuce plants. I also thought they were signs of good things to come. Worms always appeared after it rained. They came to the surface to help air and water get into the soil. I quickly learned the differences between the ants that bite and those that didn't. Bumblebees collecting pollen were attractive to me. Wasps and mosquitoes were not—especially after getting stung a few times. I was beginning to understand that all organisms have an important role in how gracefully each component of this planet will age. It is up to us to learn how we can contribute to improve and maintain our only home.

Every day provides an opportunity to unearth something new. That's where the potential rewards are. I would burst with excitement at any chance to accept nature's invitation to learn. Experience also taught me a respect for risk. At first, I perceived much more reward than risk. Time can build a healthy balance in order to preserve life. My friends and I had imaginations like sponges, soaking up all that our senses could absorb. Unlike the way I felt under the pressure of classroom tests and quizzes, I felt comfortable asking my friends the what, when, how, and why of things. There was no intimidation among friends outdoors. We were all amateur scientists testing our own theses, learning through trial and error. Unfamiliar colors, sounds, scents, textures, tastes, and feelings would command our full attention. I'd go to sleep at night, dreaming about the wonders I had witnessed. Then I'd wake up and look forward to new, future adventures. Great things happen when childlike wonder and imagination are rediscovered and combined with experience. Passion fuels these thoughts and can guide them toward actions. Life continues to teach me that youthful curiosity and discovery have no age limit. The aging process accelerates when these are no longer the center of attention.

GEMS: It's never too late to pick up a new hobby or learn new skills. It's vital to keeping the brain active and sharp. Neuroplasticity, or the creation of new connections between neurons, creates positive changes in our brains. There are many benefits waiting for us, especially when activities are done in outdoor green spaces. I've been active in nature ever since I can remember. Physical activities in an outdoor setting can help us maintain memory and reduce stress, blood pressure, and brain fog as we age. When was the last time you got some natural medicine at your local park, garden or beach?

4

SIGN OF THE TIMES: FRESHMAN FAST FOOD CHRONICLES

Why is sunset more colorful than sunrise? It's an irony of life saying, 'sometimes, good things happen in goodbyes.
— Unknown

During my freshman year of college, my appetite for fast food grew. So did my fondness for cannabis. After a few spliffs, blunts, and bong hits, my dorm mates and I would get hungry. We weren't exactly gourmet chefs, though. My culinary repertoire was limited. Eggs, sausages, spaghetti, and hot dogs got boring after a while. I went from ramen noodle novice to expert in a matter of months. I even learned how to use a skillet to fry beef burgers on the electric stove. On occasion, we'd have burger-flipping contests. The winner was determined by who could use the spatula to flip his burger the highest. Catching the burger with the spatula and safely placing it back in the grease gained points. Talk about high stakes. If your burger dropped on the dirty floor, the match was over.

The dorms were surrounded by popular chain restaurants less than a mile off campus. The food court on campus was decent but a little pricier. The dorms were located near SW 107th Avenue, an extremely busy three-lane road. The main attractions for me were Burger King, KFC, and Little Caesars Pizza. The latter had five-dollar pizza pies on Monday's. Burger King advertised frequent discounts, with signs in front of the franchise. Buy one item, get one free; ninety-nine-cent double Whoppers with cheese; free fries with a purchase, etc.—those were deals I didn't refuse. I'd combine the Whoppers with a large vanilla shake and a side of—what else?— onion rings. The closest I ever got to eating a fruit was when they ran out of vanilla shakes. I'd settle for a strawberry shake instead. That must've been lunch or dinner at least two or three times a week. I almost turned into a burger, I was such a fan of the fast-food experience. The sesame-seed buns tasted different. The beef patties we fried and fumbled in our rooms were not in the same stratosphere. The sauces and dressings that blended with the lettuce, tomato, onions, and pickles kept me coming back for more.

Shortly after hurricane Andrew wreaked havoc on South Florida, I was bored staying indoors. Classes were canceled and I hadn't cracked a book all semester. A lot of the places we used to frequent around the school were still closed due to damages. My two roommates, Charlie and Brian, were also from New York. We were all restless and agreed to venture off campus at night. We walked around and witnessed dozens of downed trees, power lines, poles, and street signs. They had been knocked down or torn loose by the storm. It was the colorful street signs that really caught our attention. We went back to the dorms and came back with pliers and a monkey wrench. What were a bunch of college students from out of state doing with those tools? Who knows? During the next few nights, we went street-sign shopping. We collected a stop sign, a one-way sign, a pedestrian-crossing sign, a Pirelli tire sign, and a yield sign—all awesome ornaments to decorate the boring-looking tan walls in our dorm room. What we came upon next made me pause and take a breath.

WILL LOISEAU

A Burger King sign was laid out on the grass. Not just a regular sign, but the huge sign that used to keep me in a trance whenever my parents drove by it when we lived in Brooklyn. I'd point the sign out to my parents each and every time we passed by. Once in a while they'd stop in either to shut me up or to satisfy their own cravings. This was the channel letter sign with the vintage red- white-and-yellow BK logo. This sign in front of us had once stood tall and brightly lit on a metal pole over the restaurant. It was visible to street traffic more than a mile away. There was also a smaller sign about fifty yards east. It used to be near the drive-thru. The larger one was the main focus. The hurricane had blown it a few hundred feet from the restaurant.

"We need this in our room, guys," I said.

"I don't think this is gonna fit, dude," said Brian, shaking his head.

"He's right. We gotta bring this back to our room tonight," Charlie said with a grin.

When we tried to lift it, we strained to hold it up. The sign was made of some type of Plexiglas and was heavy. We went back to the dorms to get more manpower. Besides, we'd have to come back later because, although it was midnight, the roads were still too busy. Carrying that huge sign across both sides of SW 107th Ave would be too risky with so many cars driving by.

We didn't have to do much convincing to get Nate and Kevin, our other comrades, to assist us. They were still up, too. We went back out to the site at 3:00 A.M. Now there were five of us. Four of us grabbed a corner and the other one guided the middle. We carried the sign about thirty yards closer to the street and dropped it on the grass when we saw cars coming. If the cops caught us, we'd probably get arrested and kicked out of school. We looked both ways, picked up the sign, and went for it again.

"One, two, three!" With small, quick steps we were off. The sign was much heavier than it appeared. It felt like it weighed hundreds of pounds. We saw a few headlights in the distance, approaching in our direction. There was no turning back now. All we could do was hope those lights weren't on a cop car. We got to the median.

"I'm losing my grip. Let's put this down for a second," Brian said.

"I feel your pain, but we gotta get this to the other side," Kevin told him.

The edges of the sign were hard, sharp, and unforgiving. The traffic light at the nearest intersection on SW Eighth Street was red, but a few headlights were lurking in the distance.

"Suck it up, man. We've got a clear lane," Charlie yelled.

My heart beat faster every time a few cars passed behind us. A few honked their horns, but none of them stopped. I tried to ignore them, but we literally looked like a bunch of deer in the headlights.

"Go, go, go!" We shuffled our feet as fast as we could as the traffic light turned green.

The edges of the sign felt sharper the longer we held it. The weight dug into our hands. We reached a grassy area on the other side of the road.

"Guys, let's put this thing down. It's killing my hands," Nate said.

With us holding the edges, most of the sign's weight drooped toward the middle. This made it difficult to hold for extended periods.

Once we got on campus, there was a slight feeling of relief. The toughest part was finally over, or so we thought. When we reached our dorm room, we set the sign down to map out an entry strategy. The sign was bigger than we'd thought. We tilted it diagonally and tried to push it through the door frame. The material the sign was made of did not bend much. We managed to push it halfway in before it got stuck.

It was now around 4:00 A.M. We were wired and waking up the building with our infectious adrenaline.

"Guys, you can't be serious. What are you doing?" Darleen, our building's resident assistant, came down the stairs from the second floor. She wore a bonnet, sweats, and slides. Her eyes were full of sleep.

"Hey, Darleen. Didn't mean to wake you up. We're just doing a little redecorating," I said with a grin.

"I can't believe what I'm seeing right now. You guys need to wrap this up as quickly as possible. If anyone files a complaint, we're all in big trouble."

"We should be done in a few minutes," I chimed in.

"I'm gonna make believe I never saw any of this." She walked away, shaking her head in disbelief.

"A few minutes? Try another hour," Nate said.

"This end is stuck in the door frame," said Kevin.

All five of us tried pulling and pushing. It wouldn't budge. After all the work we'd put in to get it here, the sign wasn't moving.

"We're going to have to remove the door," Charlie said.

"Yeah, we might have to remove this bottom plate from the floor, too," I added.

After taking off the door, it took thirty minutes of pushing, kicking, pulling, and finally pounding with a mallet to get the sign into the dorm room. None of us had imagined it would take so much effort to pull this off. If we had, we probably would have left the sign right where it was. Each dorm building had two floors. We wouldn't have tried if we had lived on the second floor.

We rearranged the furniture to make space in front of the wall outlet in the living room. The sign took up the entire wall. Nate came up with the idea of putting Christmas tree lights behind it. The sign was right next to the large sliding glass window. When we pulled up the blinds, the sign was visible to anyone who walked by. At night, we'd keep the room lights off and let the sign light up the room with a cool, dim glow. We became known around campus as the dudes with the Burger King sign. To me, the sign was the ultimate nostalgia. It was synonymous with the smell of flame-broiled burgers, the smoke blowing from the chimney, the anticipation of eating what was on the menu, and wearing the paper BK crown when celebrating my birthday with friends. This felt like a full-circle moment. The restaurant would be closed for a while longer until repairs were completed. Before they opened back up, I had to go back to the scene the next day to get the smaller sign for my room.

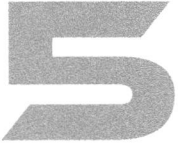

PREVENTABLE DIS-EASE: QUESTIONING CONVENTIONAL HEALTH WISDOM

An ounce of prevention is worth a pound of cure.
— *Benjamin Franklin*

The exact time and place escape my memory. But when I first heard the phrase "preventable disease," my ears perked up. This simple term suggested that I might have some type of control over my health. Instead of merely surviving disorder, it was possible to flourish. All around me people with common chronic diseases were prematurely aging. Their withering minds and bodies were mere shells of who they had been just a few years earlier. Chronic diseases were talked about ad nauseam in the media. I kept asking myself if I had unknowingly been contributing to the cause of my own issues. It seemed like everybody was suffering from something. Their symptoms kept them distracted. Sickness persisted in keeping them from enjoying the present moment. It kept us from living our best lives. I read books, watched YouTube videos, and had countless conversations with fellow practitioners in search of answers. I sought out well-respected wellness doctors domestically and abroad. I picked their brains in person, over the phone, and online. They shared their experiences in helping people free themselves from symptoms. I spotted a common theme among us. Proper nutritional science was not taught in all of the schools we attended collectively. This knowledge was nowhere in traditional curriculums. Extra time had to be applied in order to understand this area of study after graduation. I learned something new with every constructive conversation. Other times, we respectfully agreed to disagree. But one thing was clear: We were all sick and tired of living in a sick and tired society. These interactions gave me more understanding. My perception of what role I could play to make a difference became clearer.

My experience with research writing as an English major was a great skill set to have. I used internet search engines to find well-documented medical literature with solid evidence. Obesity, type 2 diabetes, strokes, hypertension, autoimmune issues, etc., were identified as largely avoidable. I discovered Dr. Otto Warburg. He won the Nobel Peace Prize in Physiology or Medicine in 1931. He claimed that 80 percent of cancers could be avoided—simply by reducing the level of carcinogens. I had never heard of carcinogens. These are substances associated with or known to cause cancer. Warburg considered this illness to be mainly a nutritional problem, one that could be avoided by maintaining a natural diet free of cancer-causing agents. This led me to read a book titled *The China Study,* by T. Colin Campbell. It explored the relationship between nutrition, heart, and metabolic diseases. I was convinced that nutrition could either feed or starve illness. Little by little, things were beginning to make sense.

I've crossed paths with many beautiful souls who passed away much earlier than I expected. The manifestations of common diseases seemed so . . . common. I kept finding confirmation that the severe symptoms I suffered from were all preventable. That's right. Asthma, bronchitis, pneumonia, boils, allergies, flus, periodontal disease, fevers, joint pains, eczema, hemorrhoids, tendonitis, and cloudy vision were all a result of the poor lifestyle choices I was making. Each horrific experience I survived was an attempt to teach me another lesson. I just didn't get it. I believed what I heard on the television, from allopathic doctors, and via word of mouth that these popular symptoms were "genetic," "hereditary," or "ran in my family." So I kept on living in a mental fog, wondering if the majority of my health outcomes were out of my control. One trait I do believe was passed on to me was the superpower of stubbornness. I just refused to believe that I was powerless against the causes of an unhealthy existence.

As the proverb says, "In the land of the blind, the one-eyed man is king."

Critical thinking wasn't encouraged in the primary and secondary schools I attended. Questioning the information being taught was treated as a disruption of the class. Skepticism regarding course materials was generally frowned upon. Deductive reasoning to form my own judgments went against the system. These unused skills were crucial, especially during the formative years of my development. Many of my classmates throughout the years eventually became parents. Naturally, they shared what they learned in school with their children. Today, prompts frequently appear on my cell phone, nudging me to update the operating system. Yet the factory-model school curriculum has not been modernized since the early nineteenth century. Generations of children, including me, have been taught to memorize answers for standardized tests. They blindly follow instructions without asking critical questions . . . just like I did. Seeking multiple opposing sources, questioning generic answers, and applying information in the real world were things I had to learn to do on my own. Teaching myself these skills allowed me to overcome years of accumulating symptoms. Contrary to what I believed, chronic disease doesn't begin in middle age. A small, albeit gradually increasing, portion of us are born with major, irreversible challenges. But my peers and I developed these issues when we were kids. That's when excess salt, sugar, cholesterol, fat, and, yes, protein began hardening our arteries. By the time we were in our twenties, plaque had already formed. I lost close friends who didn't get to celebrate reaching thirty. Years later, heart attacks and strokes would claim even more lives.

My genetic makeup, like that of everyone else, started me off on a certain path. But what if I could get off at a different exit if that path no longer served me? What if I could reset and forge a new road for myself and those who would come after me? For that reason, it was important for me to go back and examine parts of my childhood. Many of the answers were hiding in plain sight.

I think back to breakfast in school as a child. Regular and chocolate milk were mainstays since the first grade. Small cartons of sugary milk were passed around the lunchroom. On some days the kids would whisper to one another, "Don't drink the milk!"

"Why?" I would ask with a concerned voice.

"Because it's spoiled. Pass the message," they'd reply.

This rumor was always started by an overweight kid. At the time, there were only one or two overweight or obese kids among the thirty pupils in each class. They'd always end up with an extra half dozen milk cartons from those who believed the rumor. I always fell for it. I didn't understand the significance of the "best by" date stamped on the top of the carton. Little did I know that the kids who pulled those stunts represented the advent of the current obesity epidemic.

My classmates and I believed that dairy products would help us build stronger bones and teeth. Grilled cheese sandwiches with french fries were my favorite meal at lunch. I'd ask the lunch lady for an extra handful of fries every time. Individually wrapped American cheese slices were a food I craved every night before bed. Once in a while my dad would come home with a big rectangular cardboard box. Inside was a block of yellow government cheese. It was solid as a brick, but it tasted incredible.

I was addicted to dairy. Societal cues told me that cookies were better with a tall glass of milk. This was what they showed on the popular sitcoms and cartoons on television. The sports magazines I read had strong athletes wearing milk mustaches. This concept was reinforced in health class. We were told that milk was necessary to grow big and strong. Vanilla ice cream was always in the freezer at home. Boxes of Breyer's French vanilla bean and rum raisin were finished by me after two servings. Maraschino cherries were among the few fruits I ate at the time. They came in small glass jars. Drenched in bright, thick red syrup, their color was so attractive. I'd put a large spoonful over the ice cream mounds. Ice cream sandwiches and birthday cakes from Carvel were for special occasions. I didn't even like chocolate, but the crunchy chocolate crumbs that came inside those cakes were delicious. Cheese Doodles, Doritos, mac and cheese had me strung out like a fiend. Pizza was like a religion in New York. As a latchkey kid, I'd order a large pie with extra cheese from the local pizzeria after basketball practice at least once a week. Twenty minutes after the delivery person left, the pizza box would be empty.

I snacked on chocolate chip cookies, vanilla wafers, and saltines. An assortment of sugary butter cookies that came in a royal blue circular tin got me excited. My parents would always save the container to store things in. I'd search for the cookies with the red cherry in the middle and eat all of them in one day. I was convinced that Gatorade was an elixir. Michael Jordan was having so much fun drinking it in the commercials. I wanted to play basketball at the highest level, too. I watched him drink it during almost every television time-out. I liked the way it tasted, and the marketing encouraged me to believe it was beneficial. I drank it even if I wasn't being active. Corn chips, Cheetos, salt and vinegar chips, BBQ chips, and onion rings. After varsity basketball practice, my teammates and I would scarf down bags of the latter. I even came up with a theme song: "Onion rings, onion rings, nothing like the taste of onion rings, / Onion rings, onion rings tonight / When there's nothing good to eat, it's a golden crispy treat, / Onion rings, onions rings tonight!"

The last thing on my mind was a possible connection between what I was eating and symptoms of disease. We all had foods we liked and foods we didn't care for much. I gravitated toward the foods with the extravagant flavors. Occasionally, my father would share pictures of himself with the disabled kids he bused to and from school. These kids were born without the physical mobility I had. Some had paralysis of the legs. Others had paralysis of the legs and arms. It didn't seem to matter. They were gifted in unique ways and wore the happiest smiles in each photo. My dad expressed a genuine love for those kids, but I couldn't tell if he was subconsciously reminding me how fortunate I was. I didn't know what lifestyles their parents had. Nor did I consider the impact of these on their conditions. All I knew was that the kids had no control over how they got here. So what about me and the other kids who got sick each and every year? How could we take command of our health? The more I paid attention to the symptoms my parents and people around me were going through, the closer I inched toward identifying the root common causes.

The packaged foods I grew up eating weren't available when my parents were my age. The newer supermarket aisles were stocked with new lab-created experiments. We unknowingly volunteered to play the crash-test dummies. These foods were cheap, convenient, chemically addictive, easily found, widely accepted, and heavily marketed. We all thought it was harmless to eat these foods every day or every week. I didn't lose any sleep worrying about the pros or cons of the ingredients. There was a sense of trust in the system that regulated what we could eat. There was some power or authority in charge of that, right? I didn't think about long-term health implications. I was young and attracted to experiencing immediate gratification. I thought that store items couldn't be sold if they might cause me harm in any way. Health wasn't a topic I ever discussed in depth with anyone. Not until I was sick, that is. It was an unspoken understanding that eating certain foods in moderation was okay. The catchy jingles, smiling faces and personalities on television and radio, and convincing celebrity endorsements had me fooled.

I used to believe the acid reflux, flatulence, stomachaches, rashes, pimples, lactose intolerance, and dozens of other symptoms that followed the eating of certain foods were normal. My friends and I used to slide whoopee cushions under unsuspecting victims right before they sat down in class. The looks of shock and embarrassment on their faces were priceless. We'd crack jokes and laugh at the kids who tried to hide the loud, weird noises their stomachs made after eating lunch. They were harder to conceal during tests and quizzes, when the class was quiet. I'd use the fake cough method to cover up the sounds whenever my own stomach growled. It took years for me to develop a deeper understanding of the potentially serious health conditions that follow these various symptoms. My body kept giving me warning signals that I continued to ignore. I counted on over-the-counter chemicals to provide me with quick relief. I thought they would protect me against disease. The real preventative powers actually come from the chemicals released from my body during physical exercise. When I consistently produce and let go of these (endorphin) chemicals, my mood improves, and healthy immune functions flow more easily. I also gain protective power from the chemicals naturally found in ripe fruits, vegetables, nuts, seeds, and microgreens. These plant powerhouses are rich in thousands of compounds. They're like personal invites for fertile terrain and healthy bacteria to thrive in my blood and gut microbiomes, where the bulk of my complex, immune network lies. For a long time, I had no idea this was true. Plant foods are required in order to grow healthy immune system cells. The more I ate, the better my emotional, psychological, and physical health became. I never met anyone who consistently added more unrefined plants on their plate and didn't experience better health.

As I continue to mature, health becomes an unavoidable topic. Increasingly, it's becoming a lack of health that dominates conversations. I'm now amazed by how many adults are unaware of where their food comes from. We've become afraid to get our hands dirty and are disconnected from the soil. Gardening is niche in the areas where it needs to be a necessity. Unbeknownst to some, the synthetic ingredients in popular foods are harming us. Eating low-frequency foods becomes a pattern that gradually develops into a lifestyle. The lifestyle cycle can continue for generations. I wasn't able to cure any disease I had until I stopped eating the foods that caused them.

I decided that I would do everything in my power to end the cycle of preventable disease in my family. It started with the way I interact with health-care professionals. Unlearning what I had been taught about health and relearning new information was arduous. I had built up resentment against those I felt were responsible for lost time. Once I realized that was a losing battle, I began to shift my energy. I identified weaknesses in the current system and focused on using their strengths to my advantage. Medical degrees from prestigious universities are awesome. Walls with fancy framed certificates and licenses are commendable. But how do they serve me if I can't get rid of my preventable issues? I had to find ways to identify whether the person wearing the white medical lab coat was qualified to help me.

The role that the right nutrition plays in preventing disease is criminally downplayed in med schools. I once spoke with a cardiologist while she ran an EKG (electrocardiogram) on me during an annual checkup.

"Was nutrition ever part of the curriculum when you were in med school?" I asked.

"You know, Will, I don't recall taking any nutrition classes. I took biochemistry and we learned about vitamin deficiencies. But I haven't seen too many patients who suffer from those."

"Really, how long were you in school?"

"After high school . . . about fourteen years. My last three years were internal medicine training."

"Wow. Is that common?" I replied.

"Yes. During my fellowship we worked sixty, sometimes eighty hours a week. We were so busy, I barely had time to eat, let alone give nutrition much consideration."

Before I replied, I looked at her and paused. She understood the irony of what she'd just said.

"I appreciate your being honest."

"Of course. I'm noticing that my patients and I share similar symptoms. I think the food we eat and lack of movement may be the reason."

As a cardiologist on the front lines for over a decade, she treated thousands of patients with heart problems each year. All of these interactions with patients, and yet no evidence-based nutritional training. In theory, a cardiologist's job is to find the underlying cause of cardiovascular conditions. The education these specialists receive barely gives them a fighter's chance. My heart was fine, but high morbidity rates due to heart issues represented a growing problem. For longer than I've been alive, heart disease has been the leading cause of death globally. Nutrition and lifestyle were the culprits all along.

On the way home that day, I had a conversation with a middle-aged Uber driver.

Uber driver: "Hey there, how's it going?"

"I'm well. How are you?"

"I've been dealing with some real bad arthritis in my hands and knees."

"That must be painful," I replied, looking at him in the rearview mirror.

"Yes. Especially in my hands. It can be difficult to drive sometimes," he said, opening and closing his hands repeatedly, trying to increase range of motion and decrease pain.

"How do you manage?"

"I try to stretch before and after each drive. I also take some over-the-counter medication for the pain when it gets really bad. It's hard to find the time to move, with all the driving I do."

"Have you ever looked for a professional who helps cure arthritis?"

"No . . . I never thought to get another doctor's opinion."

"No?"

"I never knew that there was a cure. My doctor said that because my father and grandfather had it, it was in my genes."

"I know. Both my parents have it, too," I replied.

"And you don't? What did you do?"

"I remembered how curious I was as a kid. For some reason, I'd stopped asking questions when I got older."

"I was always told to follow doctor's orders, so I did."

"Same here. But today there's more information available. Some good, some bad. I'm more proactive now."

"You ask more questions now?"

"Yes. As many as possible."

"Maybe I need to ask more questions, too. If I'm taking these pills, right?"

"That's right. I'd wanna know how they're supposed to help me. What risks come with putting certain chemicals in my body. When I can reduce the dosage. How can I be free from them entirely."

"No matter what I take, the pain always comes back. Do you take anything?"

"I take plants every day. Fruits and veggies eliminated my inflammation."

"I know I don't eat enough."

"You have any kids?"

"Yes, a girl. You?"

"Not yet. But if my daughter wanted to excel in a profession, I would avoid the schools with no track record of producing successful professionals. Make sense?"

"Yes," he replied, as if a lightbulb had just turn on in his mind.

"Health professionals with experience in how to cure certain conditions give me more confidence," I said, opening the door as we reached my destination.

"I'm so glad we had this conversation, Will. I have a lot to talk about with my family and my doctor.

Creating a game plan has helped me take control over my health throughout the years. I was always told as an adult to make sure to visit my doctor on a regular basis. A visit just to visit started making less sense. It was as important to know specifically what I wanted to get out of each visit. A routine checkup is maintenance. Being diagnosed with a particular illness these days requires more research by the patient and an effort to get additional professional opinions.

I marvel at the number of online videos, documentaries, books, and research materials available. Some of these books are written by well-established medical doctors. These doctors have taken the initiative to study nutritional science and have helped their patients cure common illnesses. There are numerous books I have yet to read. I've found that reaching out to people on social media groups has been helpful. People in these groups are happy to share their success stories on how they overcame their respective illnesses. A community that can sympathize with common struggles and support recovery is valuable.

I spoke with people who struggled with type 2 diabetes for years. They reversed this by changing their eating habits. I read studies that identified excess saturated fat in the diet as the main cause of this disease. Fat prevents sugar in the blood from entering muscle and liver cells. The sugar has nowhere to go. So the blood-sugar levels shoot up. I always thought sugar was the main cause. Several doctors I've met were not aware of these studies. Who knows how many of them are still telling their patients that there's no cure for type 2 diabetes? These interactions taught me a lot about the responsibilities I had. Getting additional opinions from open-minded professionals is a must. I got better at identifying those who were not open to new information. Once I began to notice the questions I was not being asked during doctors' visits, my understanding of the system totally changed. I was never asked any in-depth questions about my exercise habits. Not one doctor has ever asked for a detailed description of my diet. Discussions on the topic of sleep have been minimal at best. Did we ever discuss stress solutions? No. There was never a mention of how much time I spend outdoors. I wasn't asked any of these questions. I've since cut all ties with health-care providers who offer only experimental chemicals as a solution.

> **GEMS:** There are many options available to expedite healing preventable dis-ease. The first step for me was to unlearn and relearn most of what schools had taught me about health. As challenging as this was, it was well worth my time. I began to understand that self-care is the real health care. Everything else is a variation of alternative medicine.

Fresh plant foods, meditation, yoga, audio therapy, aroma therapy, exercise, massage, and other activities have become vital components of my self-care routine. It's up to each individual to try a variety of activities. Naturally, the mind and body will gravitate to the ones that feel best.

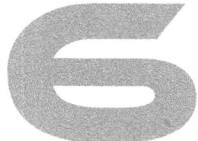

CATCHING A COLD: UNLEARNING AND RELEARNING HEALTH

Believe only your own experience. There is no fact like a fact learned from your own life.
— *Aristotle*

Dr. Llaila Afrika wrote in his book *African Holistic Health,* "A 'cold' is developed, not caught. You cannot 'catch healthy' by standing near a healthy person. You cannot catch a cold by contracting some strange bacteria or dead cell particle called a virus. A dis-eased (toxic) weakened body has little defense against a strange bacterium and is the perfect septic environment to multiply. The catarrh (mucous) discharge called a 'cold' is the body's attempt to rid itself of waste (toxic impurities) that it could not pass out through the bowels (manure) or urine or perspiration. It is usually caused by constipation, overeating or a diet of partial foods (junk foods) that produces partial health known as a disease. The body is not 'at-ease,' it is in a state of 'dis-ease' called a 'cold.'"

WILL LOISEAU

For as long as I can remember, I believed that all flus, fevers, colds, etc., were unavoidable. I was taught that germs on doorknobs, tables, and other surfaces were just waiting to be touched and make unfortunate victims sick. Whenever another person coughed or sneezed without covering their mouth, airborne particles were released into the air. Schoolteachers told my fourth-grade classmates and me that these particles could potentially travel across rooms and throughout buildings. We would then become defenseless against whatever disease that person might have had. It wasn't something I questioned, because the same theory was echoed wherever I went.

It had rained heavily for hours one autumn night on Long Island. The next morning warmed up to a crisp fifty degrees. I was running late for school, so I scarfed down some sausages and hard-boiled eggs before heading out the door. As I ran down the hill on Farrington Avenue, I came upon a small river. Not really, but the water had to have been at least two feet deep in the middle of the road. The storm drains on both sides of the road always got clogged whenever it rained hard. Normally, I'd just walk off to the side, where the grassy edge met the fence that bordered the Blackman family's front yard. The water there was shallower but appeared to be deeper than normal on this day. Pressed for time, I was trying to beat the bus to the bus stop. With my book bag on my back, I tried to get a running start, but the slippery mud made me think otherwise. From a standing position, I leaped off one foot about three yards in the air. Splashhh!!! Both feet landed in the water. I took another leap to get to the other side and splashed again. I got to the bus stop at the same time the bus arrived. I sat near the middle of the bus and looked at my feet. My pants were wet and my socks were soaked. On the bus, I emptied the water from my shoes onto the floor. I then laced them back up to enter the school. I kept those socks on my feet for all my classes. Later that night, I began to have chills and labored to breathe. I felt really sick and shook with muscle pain throughout the night.

My condition only worsened the next morning. My parents decided to take me to South Side University Hospital, a few miles away in Bay Shore. The doctors' discussion made me more anxious. They said I'd have to spend the night under their supervision. I found myself confined to a hospital bed, which was the last place I wanted to be. Later that evening, my older brother came up to stay with me after my parents left. As sick as I was, nothing could prevent me from watching my favorite performer's prime-time television appearance. My eyes were glued to the television screen that night to watch Motown's twenty-fifth-anniversary special. Michael Jackson put on a solo performance that shook up the entertainment industry. I was in awe when he moonwalked across the stage. Despite the limited media coverage of such events at that time compared to today, I sensed his longing to recapture the childhood experiences that the demands of show business had denied him.

The next morning a doctor diagnosed me with severe pneumonia. What I thought would be a one-night stay ended up being more than a week. My chest hurt with each breath. I couldn't keep any food in my stomach. The only reaction my body had toward food was either vomiting or diarrhea. It was up to my lungs to eliminate the accumulation of toxins in my body. It was daily doses of hospital food and prescription chemicals unless my parents brought me some home-cooked food. Apart from Michael's iconic performance, I was miserable for most of the time. I was allowed to go home after my body stopped rejecting food and liquids.

My mom refused to let the situation rest, though. She swore I got sick because I kept wet socks on my feet. Was that the real reason I came close to losing my life as a teen? Not exactly. Wearing wet socks for a whole day wasn't the most brilliant idea. But that couldn't be the only reason I ended up in the hospital. Coughing, sneezing, and blowing my nose were common activities for me and lots of other kids. These were the ways my body chose to rid itself of mucus. But where did the mucus come from? I had to have made mucus as a response to the foods I was eating. Chicken, white rice, dairy products, beef, breakfast cereals, candy, fast food, potato chips, soda and other sugary drinks were the norm for me. No one around me was aware that these were mucus-forming foods. My body produced mucus to envelope the incoming toxins and encourage an evacuation response. Stepping into a puddle of muddy water was where my body finally reached its tipping point. I couldn't interpret the warning signs and indicators my system was sending. It had been communicating with me through allergic reactions, colds, flus, aches and pains, fevers, headaches, diarrhea, and stomachaches. All of those symptoms were internal protests against what I was putting in my mouth. The pneumonia was my body's way of conducting an emergency shutdown. In order to remove the buildup of toxins, I had to be forced into an extended period of rest.

During the hospital stay, I blamed myself for keeping the socks on. I must have been told dozens of times not to play in the rain because I'd get sick. This was reinforced as the only conclusion, according to my parents and other family members. Why? They were taught some similar version in the schools they attended. This was what was regurgitated over and over. Decades later, allopathic medical school students are not taught anything different. The naturopathic philosophy that I later discovered taught the exact opposite of everything I had been absorbing for decades. Imagine unlearning and relearning everything you knew about health well into adulthood. I have accepted that doing so will be a lifelong process. These days, I regularly run miles outdoors in the rain. Depending on the sneakers I'm wearing, I might even look for puddles to splash my feet in.

I used to wonder why whenever one person in a class, office, or household got sick, other dominoes would begin to fall. Is there a correlation? *Merriam-Webster's* defines the word *correlation* as the relationship between things that happen or change together. When I revisited what my classmates, coworkers, and family members usually had in common, one pattern began to stick out.

I'd notice the more time we spent with one another, the more we shared similar habits.

I likened this to two houses in different parts of town. Let's call them House A and House B. House A is not a very healthy place to be. It's filled with salty fast foods, mind-altering narcotics, hard alcohol, thick cigarette smoke, loud, profanity-laced music, accumulating trash, and a really dirty bathroom with a slow, stinky, stagnant cesspool. On the other hand, House B is a much better place to live. It has fresh fruit and vegetable spreads, fresh flowers, meditation zones, and a clean bathroom with a free-flowing waste-management system. These two houses are completely different. If we think of the people living in each house, those in House A would face a lot of potential problems. It's like a dangerous trap waiting to cause trouble. On the other hand, the people in House B would have a better chance at healthier possibilities. They would feel more comfortable in their environment the longer they stayed there.

Before I learned about taking care of myself, I spent a long time in a House A kind of environment. It was what I knew and was used to. But then I realized that I had the power to control the kind of environment I created for myself, both internally and externally. Taking care of my body has gradually become more of a priority for me. It's influenced by the kind of food I eat, how much exercise I get, the quality of sleep I have, how much sunlight my skin gets, the quality of air I breathe, and even the quality of my thoughts. All of these things play a role in how well my body can protect itself and stay healthy. Now here's an interesting question: If the people from both houses were all born in the same year, who would look younger over time? Would it be the people from House A or House B?

Living in New York for most of my life, I got to see how my behavior could change with the seasons. Each autumn, the clock got pushed back one hour for daylight saving time. I love the sun. Knowing the days would be getting shorter made the fall and winter my least favorite times of year. It was dark and gloomy when I got up before 7:00 A.M. to go to work. The sun would set around the time I got out of work around 4:00 P.M. This had such a powerful psychological effect. It was disorienting, and I found myself feeling more tired and less motivated than usual.

No bright rays to greet me in the morning made me not want to get out of bed on most days. No sunshine in the evening made me want to go to bed earlier. I usually stayed indoors more to keep warm. Being inside closed environments had me breathing more recycled air. The more hours spent breathing artificially heated air blown through dirty air vents only increased opportunities to get sick. More time inside also meant less exposure to the sun, the brightest mood booster I know. I had an increased desire for eating comfort junk foods. I saw them as allies in avoiding depression and negative mood swings. Most of these foods had to be heated. Since I couldn't get warmth from the sun, heating up food was an attempt to warm up my insides.

A repetitive theme from coworkers at just about any job I ever had was, "I can't do anything without my hot chocolate or cup of coffee!" or "I need at least two cups of coffee to stay awake for this meeting." Their dependency on caffeinated drinks was due to lack of sleep. As an adolescent, I slept eight to nine hours and napped almost daily. Now adults wore imaginary badges of honor for not sleeping. I've only seen chronic insomnia lead to more problems—lack of productivity, irritability, and increased susceptibility to illness, just to name a few. I noticed that the older people got, the less they were exposed to fresh air, sunlight, good sleep, and physical activity. As a kid, I would play outside when it got cold. I'd take in deep breaths of cold winter air and play outside for hours. I didn't rebreathe stale air with germs from other people. I built snow castles, snowmen, snow angels, and, of course, had snowball fights, which were mandatory activities in my neighborhood. As long as I was dressed properly and in motion, I gave myself chances to improve my immune system. As an adult, I've noticed a change. The colder the temperatures get outside, the more we neglect our health. This is especially true during the holiday season. The focus turns to indulging in material things to stay in the "holiday spirit." I, too, engaged in increased alcohol consumption, drug use, reckless spending, and bouts of depression. My body's ability to keep me immune soon became compromised by maintaining unhealthy practices. Lack of immunity was why I and others around me got sick during the flu season. It's why I got sick whenever I encountered anyone or anything that posed the slightest threat to my health. My daily hygiene habits, no matter what season it was, had a major influence on whether I was able to maintain natural immunity.

It became strikingly clear why staying healthy was such a challenge. Western lifestyle habits only exacerbated my genetic predispositions. Implementing lifestyle changes at an aggressive yet manageable pace allowed my natural immunity to thrive in ways I used to only imagine. It's no longer a mystery to me why disease outbreaks occur so often. This is happening increasingly among humans. Other times, it's the animals we encounter that suffer and that we should probably distance ourselves from. The inevitable unfamiliar virus variants that ensue cause panic among the masses. I can't remember a time when I was able to make clear judgments when consumed by fear. This state of mind can build debilitating levels of stress. It also ages the body considerably. By showing more acts of kindness to myself and others, I can help improve my local and global environment. A cleaner climate is more conducive to the well-being of all life on this planet.

> **GEMS:** Unfortunately, I and many others around the world do not grow 100 percent of the food we eat. Foods labeled as organic can be too expensive for many people. Conventionally grown produce is heavily sprayed with chemicals that can have costly consequences with regard to our health. Eliminating all of these chemicals may not be possible. Some of these chemicals are absorbed through the outer layer of produce. Before I eat such foods, I soak them in a homemade white vinegar and baking soda solution for ten minutes. After rinsing them with warm

water, I may even scrub lightly with a gentle brush. I've found this effective in removing most of the pesticide chemicals.

THE ILLUSION OF LABELS: THE HIDDEN REALITIES BEHIND TITLES

> *If everything had a label, we would live in a fully delineated but false world.*
> — *Mason Cooley*

When I moved to Arizona for school, something happened that made me start thinking differently about what I eat. I had just finished a college class and was looking for a place to eat before my next class. That's when I ran into two classmates who were also leaving class. They were going to grab a bite to eat and invited me to join them. As we walked, we talked about what kind of food we should get. That's when they told me they didn't eat meat. I was surprised, because I thought adults needed to eat meat to be healthy. But these guys were fit, full of energy, and definitely not malnourished. So I asked them why they didn't eat meat.

They explained that animal foods can have negative effects on our health. It immediately made sense to me. They encouraged me to look into the hormones and chemicals that are given to farm animals and how our bodies respond after eating them. We ended up at a Mexican restaurant nearby. They ordered bean burritos with guacamole, and I did the same. I felt good afterward, despite not eating meat. It was the first time I had gone to a restaurant and skipped meat. I didn't completely stop eating meat that day. I thought about it for months, actually, but it wasn't long after that I proudly called myself a "vegetarian." It felt like a cool choice that would help me take care of my health and avoid the chronic diseases I saw affecting so many people around me. I was searching for answers, and being vegetarian seemed like a clear solution.

However, as time went by, I discovered that labels and titles can be misleading. I hardly ever ate any vegetables. And when I did, they were so processed that they didn't even look like vegetables anymore, and were devoid of any nutritional value. It took me years to truly understand the impact of my choices and where my food came from. I began to understand that plants are like chemical factories that produce almost all the nutrients my body needs. Years later, I came across videos that exposed the immense suffering animals endure within the confines of factory farming. That didn't sit right with my love for other animals.

But my journey to a plant-only diet was not without its challenges. When I wasn't eating burritos, I was consuming meal-replacement shakes every single day, ignoring the long list of ingredients on the label and focusing only on the protein content. Many of those ingredients were not beneficial to better health. I wasn't eating any leafy green vegetables, fruits, or sprouts, and the only nuts and seeds I consumed were in the form of processed granola bars. I still felt great because of what I was no longer consuming, but I was in my mid-twenties, and a lot of deficiencies can hide underneath the surface at that age.

At that time, there were no YouTube videos to help guide me. Today, however, there are plenty of articles, videos, and public figures paid by sponsors, institutions, and corporations to spread misinformation, leaving the average person looking for healthy choices lost and confused. I heard personal trainers at the gym tell their clients they needed to buy all types of synthetic supplements. Numerous doctors have told me that I needed some type of animal protein in my life for iron and vitamin B_{12}. Today, fit-looking social media influencers are always selling cookbooks filled with recipes on how to make gooey chocolate protein pancakes with marshmallows. Convincing until the public becomes aware that behind the scenes, they're suffering from the same health issues as their followers.

Despite the challenges, I consider myself a health foodie. I take pleasure in visiting vegan restaurants in every city I travel to, even though they don't always serve the healthiest food. Maybe it's because I remember when there were no vegan eateries. In many cases, however, they are healthier than eating at the known fast-food staples, and they offer me the opportunity to indulge in familiarity and move on, thus keeping me from craving the junk foods I used to eat.

In Western culture, dining out is the popular way to commemorate almost any occasion. During one such celebration with my work colleagues, I found myself facing a menu with very few options I could eat. I had been focusing on continuing the improvements I felt from consuming whole foods. The only dish I could identify as edible was the house salad. Shortly after, our orders arrived, and as the servers presented the dishes, I sensed all gazes fixed on my plate. To my delight, it showcased a vivid spectrum of greens, reds, oranges, yellows, and purples, which left others somewhat perplexed.

Everyone noticed there was no meat on it. One coworker said, "Wow. That's beautiful. Are you a vegetarian or vegan?'

"No. I just love to eat plants," I replied.

"Isn't that vegan?"

"Sure. Vegans don't eat animals, either . . . mainly for ethical reasons."

"So you don't eat any meat?"

"No, I feel so much better when I just eat plants."

"I commend your discipline. I love meat way too much to ever do that."

I understood the need to use titles to organize people. It's a way to make sense of things in our minds. The word *vegan* describes what a person does not eat. It says nothing about what an individual actually eats. I didn't have animal welfare in mind when I decided to stop eating them. I wasn't opposed to wearing leather belts and shoes. I didn't feel self-conscious about owning a car with leather seats. I may have even had a few leather jackets in my closet. I showed no animosity toward dogs, cats, or any other pets. I stopped eating dead animals for health reasons. I finally figured out that going against my anatomical design by eating them was causing friends, family members, coworkers, and myself to experience debilitating dis-ease or premature death. I also began to realize there were levels of health that most vegans, let alone the majority of the meat-eating population, were not achieving.

For years, I held the belief that a whole food lifestyle was only for wealthy or middle-class people, and that it was ultra-expensive and unattainable. And while there is some truth to that, as most people in the world live on less than two dollars per day, I have also come to realize that the price of something and its value are not always the same. Walking up and down the aisles of health food stores in developed countries like the United States, I estimate that at least 80 percent of chain store shelves are filled with overpriced junk. I felt like I was paying more for the packaging than the quality of the actual food. Meanwhile, street vendors in countries we call "Third World" sell fresh local produce at a fraction of the cost, picked at peak ripeness and with more nutrients, thanks to soil that is less damaged from excess toxic chemicals.

What I've also learned is that the processed products on store shelves have gone through high-temperature cooking, leading to free radical–laden proteins called advanced glycation end products (AGEs), which have been known to cause premature aging. I've had to educate myself on the major difference between minimally processed, fresh, living plant foods, and ultra-processed foods given a vegetarian or vegan label. I've spoken with many business owners of vegan foods companies who don't practice a vegan lifestyle. On the other hand, living plants from nature have a life force that helps to transform every cell in the body in magical ways.

Some of the best produce I've ever tasted has come from my very own garden. I've become obsessed with perfecting the composition of the soil, experimenting with dense soil for colder climates and sandy soil for tropical zones. It's amazing how much difference the soil can make in the taste and quality of the plants I grow. I've also learned that the timing of when I pick the produce is crucial to ensure maximum flavor and nutrient content.

Unlike the commercial produce that travels long distances and is picked unripe, my homegrown fruits and vegetables are free from harmful pesticides and other chemicals. I'm always cautious about consuming food that isn't homegrown, knowing that corporate interests often prioritize profits over health. It's disheartening to know that a handful of corporate institutions own the majority of farmland and water rights in the United States, and I worry about the impact this has on the availability of fresh and healthy food for everyone, especially those who are underserved.

One thing that has struck me is how people often identify themselves with their health conditions, such as claiming to be a "type 2 diabetic" or a "cancer survivor." It's concerning to see how these titles can become ingrained in their minds, shaping their perception of themselves and their capabilities to heal. Many of them believe that there's little they can do to overcome their health challenges, and they've been misled by misconceptions about certain foods, such as fruit sugar causing diabetes.

In reality, it's the interconnected nutrients found in fruits and other whole foods that can actually help eliminate the symptoms of type 2 diabetes. It's the saturated fat from unhealthy food choices that is the true culprit behind this disease, but that's often overlooked. Similarly, many cancers are caused by poor diet and lifestyle choices, but having a tumor removed and being in remission doesn't necessarily mean being truly cancer-free.

I vividly remember a holiday gathering where food was the centerpiece, as it often is. While others indulged in meats, salads, cakes, and snacks, I opted for a healthy salad made from fresh vegetables. A family member offered me some "light salad dressing," but upon reading the label, I knew that it was far from healthy. The list of ingredients was filled with processed substances and items with unpronounceable names, a stark contrast to the natural and nutrient-rich vegetables in my salad. It made me realize how corporations prioritize appearance, smell, and taste over the health of consumers.

Throughout this journey, I've come to realize the power of words and labels. While they can help categorize subjects, they can also be misleading when used without proper context. I've learned to question and investigate the true meaning of terms to make informed choices. After all, my priority is my health, and I strive to align my choices with that goal, supporting local farmers, promoting farming communities, and constantly learning about different plants and nutrition. In a world where food shortages and clean water issues continue to plague underserved communities, it's now more important than ever to prioritize our health and be mindful of the choices we make when it comes to our nutrition. I've learned that the best produce is the one I grow myself, nourished by the rich soil I've carefully cultivated and free from harmful chemicals. It's a labor of love, a pursuit of true health, and a constant quest for knowledge and wisdom in understanding the impact of our choices on our bodies and our overall well-being.

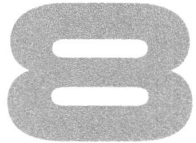

SELF-MEDICATION: MANEUVERING LIFE IN A HAZE OF INTOXICATION

Go easy on yourself. Whatever you do today, let it be enough.
— *Anonymous*

Returning to Long Island from Arizona was a pivotal moment in my journey—one that forced me to confront the inner demons that had been plaguing me. As I made my way back to the place I had always known as home, I found myself struggling to adjust to a new reality. In the nearly four years that I was away, I had undergone a transformation. I grew out my hair and had braids, stopped eating meat, lost weight, read the Quran daily, and had gone through other changes that were essential to my growth. But when I returned home, many of the people I knew had moved away or were in different stages of their lives, leaving me feeling like I was starting over.

It was like trying to patch my life back together. I couldn't help but feel like I was behind in life, as if I had not accomplished what my peers had. I struggled with feelings of inadequacy and self-doubt as I tried to adjust. But I knew that I had to keep moving forward and trust the journey.

As I reintegrated into life back home, I realized that the person I had become in Arizona was not the person I wanted to be on Long Island. I needed to find a way to integrate my new identity with my old one, to create a version of myself that felt authentic and true to who I was. It was a challenging process, but it was also a necessary one. And as I navigated the obstacles, I began to understand that confronting my inner demons was the key to unlocking a more fulfilling life.

My decision to go back to school was motivated mostly by a desire to finish what I had started. My college journey had been tumultuous, to say the least. I had been in and out of school for several years, with little progress to show for my efforts. A few years prior, a counselor at Arizona State University had pointed out that English was the only class where I never received a grade lower than a C. Was this a sign that I was overlooking a talent that needed to be explored further? Writing had always been a passion of mine, but I had never considered pursuing it as a career. I'd earned an associate's degree in liberal arts from Farmingdale State but didn't make much use of it. Now I was nervous about how many of my college credits would transfer to a new school.

I applied to Stony Brook University, a local school with a strong academic reputation, and was surprised to be accepted despite the fact that my transcripts showed several Ds and Fs. It made me wonder whether the university system was more concerned with the revenue it generated than with the academic aptitude of its students. I scheduled an appointment to visit the counselor's office to discuss my academic plan. The counselor informed me that with my current credits, I could finish a bachelor's degree in a year and a half if I was willing to take on eighteen-credit semesters. The idea of finishing my degree quickly was appealing, and I ended up taking out loans to cover the cost of classes, books, room, and board. However, as someone who had not lived on campus since my freshman year at Florida International University, I was apprehensive about living with younger students. I was a different person now, and I didn't know how to navigate being an older student on campus. I kept reminding myself that it was a means to accomplishing a greater goal, and that I needed to keep pushing forward.

Settling into a new routine wasn't easy. It was challenging not to compare myself to others and wonder if I had made the right decision to pursue a four-year degree. It was easier to immerse myself in textbooks and papers than to face the realities of the world outside. At times, I wasn't sure if I was using school as a way to hide from off-campus life or if I genuinely wanted to be there.

I took a calculated risk as the fall semester began, challenging myself by taking on more credits than I ever had before. This time, I had exclusively literary courses on my schedule, with no math or science to worry about—the subjects that had previously caused me to receive non-passing grades. If I stayed focused for the entire sixteen-week semester, I could move one-third of the way closer to the finish line. Back in Arizona, I had experienced periods of time when I would spend months voluntarily reading books and working on creative writing for most of the day. It was an immersive experience that allowed me to dive deep into my studies, but it was also isolating.

When I arrived at Stony Brook, I was placed in the Irving dorm, one of the Mendelsohn Quad buildings. Unfortunately, the school was behind schedule in completing the new dorm buildings, so they had to pack three students per room in spaces that were meant for two. I found myself sharing a small room with two other guys. There was one bunk bed and one single bed, and we had two desks and two closets to share. As an only child who met my half-siblings later in life, this was new to me. The only bunk beds I'd ever seen were on television. Willis and his little brother, Arnold, shared one on the sitcom *Diff'rent Strokes*. The school told us that this arrangement would only be temporary, but I couldn't believe this was real. The other two guys and I settled the matter of who would get the single bed with a coin toss. I ended up on the top bunk, which I thought was better than the bottom, but it was not at all what I'd expected.

In order to make ends meet, I kept my side job selling satellite dish programming door-to-door. It was a hustle, but if I put in the effort, I could consistently earn $150 in just a couple of hours. I tried to stay busy and out of the dorm as much as possible, returning only to shower or sleep. Even keeping occupied, I struggled adjusting to earlier sunsets than I'd gotten used to. In Arizona, it was hot nearly year-round, minus a few December weeks. As the weather cooled down in the East, I found myself missing the dry heat that I had grown accustomed to.

On top of that, I couldn't help but notice that I was surrounded by students who were younger than I was. It was a stark contrast to my experiences in the past, where I had always been among the youngest in my peer group. I tried not to let it bother me, but the thought of being the old man on campus weighed heavily on my mind. As a freshman, I remember how my friends and I poked fun at the students who were several years older than we were; I never imagined that one day I would be in their shoes. It seemed like nature's way of evening the score.

The campus was bustling with activity in the day, and it was hard not to feel like an outsider. As I walked to class, I couldn't help but feel like everyone was staring at me, judging me for being an older student who didn't quite fit in. I attended every class and took good notes. Whether I ever reviewed what I wrote down in class was another story. I was a master procrastinator when it came to writing papers and completing assignments. When they piled up, I'd tackle them at the last minute. It wasn't always easy, but I put in enough work to pass. Still, doubts crept in from time to time. Was I really cut out for this? Was I wasting my time? It was a constant battle to push those thoughts aside and focus on the present moment, to remind myself of why I was there in the first place.

As the end of the semester approached and finals loomed, I couldn't help but feel like I was falling behind my peers. I was far from making the dean's list, but at least I was passing all of my classes. I was performing better than in my previous attempts at college, but it still didn't feel like enough. I needed assurance that I was still on track, so I arranged a follow-up appointment with the counselor. I thought I had a good idea of what classes I needed to take in order to graduate, but the counselor had some different news for me.

After reviewing my transcripts, the counselor told me that I would need to complete an extra semester. I was devastated. It was hard to contain my anger and disappointment as I held back the urge to leap over the desk and unleash fists and feet of fury. This wasn't the carefree college experience that I had envisioned when I first arrived on campus. I wasn't having fun anymore, and the fact that I was now an adult living on my own with the financial burden of paying for an extra semester frustrated me. My student loan debt would only be deferred for a limited amount of time. Physically, I was back home, but mentally, I was in a foreign territory. It felt like I was on a long business trip, and I wasn't sure where I was going. Writing had always allowed me to time-travel to the past and suspend time in the present, but I wasn't sure how it fit into my future anymore. Leaving the counselor's office that day, my outlook on everything had changed.

The campus was sprawling, boasting nearly twenty thousand enrolled students. Despite its size, it was mainly a commuter campus, and the parking lots were constantly overflowing with cars. Some people even required shuttle buses to ferry them to and from their vehicles. By 4:59 p.m. every weekday, the lots would be nearly empty as students, faculty, and state employees made their way home. Even the on-campus kids disappeared on weekends. As for me, I struggled to fit in, feeling self-conscious about my age and like I was walking around with a sign on my back that read 27 and still in college.

I didn't anticipate living with roommates who were experiencing college for the first time. Most of them were fresh out of high school, still living with their parents, and hadn't yet faced the harsh realities of life outside of academia. Meanwhile, my own life experiences had taken me on a different path. While my high school peers were settling down, getting advanced degrees, buying homes, starting families, and building their careers, I was still figuring out who I was and where I wanted to go. I'd led a nomadic life, bouncing from state to state and school to school, and now that sense of rootlessness made it difficult for me to connect with others on campus. I felt like an outsider, lost in my own thoughts and unsure of where to turn. One day I was working at my part-time job; the next day I was hustling to record rap demo CDs in the hopes of making it on the radio. I had no clear direction for my future, and that lack of focus made me feel even more disconnected.

After the school relocated students into bigger rooms, I was left with just one roommate, who wasn't very social. Our interactions were awkward at best. I was losing interest in attending classes and didn't want to be around anyone. To ease my stress, I started smoking more marijuana, even increasing my intake to heighten that feeling of escape. As a former distributor, it was easy for me to find what I was looking for on campus, and what started out as a twenty-dollar-a-week fix quickly became a much more expensive habit. I turned to alcohol, using it as a crutch to numb the pain and escape reality. I started taking a couple shots of hard liquor before my morning classes. It wasn't long before my drinking spiraled out of control, and I found myself in a dark place. The weight of my depression felt overwhelming, and I wasn't sure how to move forward.

As the days grew colder, I found myself struggling more and more. But there was one thing that brought me a small measure of comfort: the hot showers in the dorms. The scalding water was almost unbearable when turned up to the max, but I found myself drawn to it nonetheless. It was as if the heat that tapped into a part of my senses was different from the heat of the sun. As the water cascaded over me, I closed my eyes and allowed myself to be transported to another place—a place where I felt in control, and where the uncertainties of my new life couldn't reach me.

The shower stall became a sanctuary for me—a place to reflect on the mental obstacles I was trying to overcome. I stood there, my skin turning red from the heat, and allowed myself to confront the deep sense of loneliness and depression that had settled over me. The water was a balm for my wounded soul, and I stayed there until the last drop of hot water ran out.

One day, Donte, a kid from the football team whom I had bought weed from a few times, invited me to a party. I usually kept to myself and never attended any of the school functions, but Monte seemed cool and promised that there would be girls there. We hung out together for a while, smoked a blunt and drank some cognac out of Solo cups. I planned to return to my room to eat, shower, and change before returning in an hour or so to head off to the party.

However, after stepping out of the steaming shower, I began to notice something: My skin was starting to suffer. I looked into the mirror and was shocked by what I saw. My face was red and swollen all over. My skin was sensitive to the touch and I realized that I had pushed it too far. The scalding water was stripping away my natural oils, leaving me dry and itchy. I was unknowingly trying to compensate for my emotional discomfort with a physical one, and it was taking a toll. I quickly washed my face with cold water and slathered it with lotion, hoping to reduce the swelling. But my efforts were in vain. As I stared at my reflection in the mirror, I knew that I would miss the party. Donte and I didn't have each other's contact info. That was the last time I ever saw him.

As I woke up on Monday morning, I still felt inflammation on my face and body. It was as if my skin were screaming out, begging for help. But I couldn't skip class—not when I was already skating on thin ice because of my grades. I rummaged through my closet, searching for anything that could conceal the redness and swelling. But there was nothing. Just a full bottle of vodka, tempting me with its promise of temporary relief. I knew it was a slippery slope, but I couldn't resist. I took a shot, hoping it would dull the pain and make the day pass by more quickly. I even rinsed my mouth with mouthwash, hoping I could hide the stench of alcohol from my classmates and professors. And just in case I might appear too high, I took a few hits of weed to balance out the alcohol.

Slinking into the back row of each class, I sat there like a ghost. My mind was a million miles away, lost in a haze of intoxication. I was barely hanging on, struggling to keep up with the professor's words and stay conscious. The only reason I showed up was to avoid getting zeros on the quizzes, which served as proof of attendance. I knew it wasn't a sustainable plan, but at that moment, it was all I had.

This self-medication quickly became a costly habit. I was spending hundreds of dollars a month on alcohol and weed. I had minimal contact with family and friends and felt myself sinking deeper into depression. I became a functioning addict, only leaving my room to stumble to class or get food. This went on for months, until the semester ended.

The icy grip of winter had held me in its clutches for far too long. My depression had only grown worse as I isolated myself in my dorm room, drowning my issues in bottles and smoke. But as the temperature began to rise, something shifted inside of me. I decided to take a chance and venture out of my room, heading to the campus gym a few times a week. It was there that I started to meet new people—young, vibrant students who shared my love of exercise. We played pickup basketball or lifted weights together, and I found myself enjoying their company. I was drawn to their energy and enthusiasm for life. It was contagious, and it began to rub off on me. During my last semester, I even started dating a girl I had met in one of my English classes. We were paired up in a group project, and I found myself smiling more when I was around her.

While I didn't completely quit drinking and smoking, I started to slow down considerably. The more time I spent socializing, the easier it became to pull myself away from my destructive tendencies. I no longer felt the need to escape from who I was. Slowly but surely, I was making my way back. I was heading in the right direction.

Looking back on that time in my life, I realize that I was not in a healthy place. But at the time, it was all I knew how to do to deal with my emotions. I was seeking temporary comforts to cover deep wounds. Some required more time to heal than others. I would have told my younger self that it was okay to be on a different path and that my worth was not determined by my age or academic achievements. I now realize that my experience was not uncommon. Many older students struggle with feeling out of place on campus, questioning their abilities and their place in the world. Living in a dormitory full of teenagers and young twentysomethings may not have been what I expected, but in a strange way it was what I needed. Their passion for learning and exploration was contagious. They taught me that you become old once you stop learning new things. Besides, today's online courses make learning at home much easier. But it's important to remember that everyone's journey is unique, and success is not always measured in the same way. My anxieties were all in my head. I had to learn to let go of the comparisons and focus on my own path to success, one step at a time.

> **GEMS:** At the time of this writing, it has been decades since I've taken a hot shower. In that time, I discovered cold showers. Some of the benefits I've experienced are reduced inflammation, especially after running long distances and other intense training. My skin has a more youthful complexion too. I was prematurely aging my skin with the harmful hot water. Cold water also helps to reduce stress. The initial shock influences the release of stress hormones which activate my parasympathetic nervous system. This slows down the heart rate, lowers blood pressure, and promotes better digestion.

WILL LOISEAU

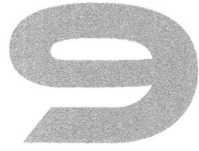

CHANGE: THE EMAIL THAT ALTERED MY PATH

Change will not come if we wait for some other person or some other time. We are the ones we've been waiting for. We are the change that we seek.
— Barack Obama

Not long after I returned from the massive earthquake in Haiti, the bank I was working at decided to move forward with their plans to relocate from New York to Virginia. Being a bookkeeper didn't inspire me, nor did it benefit my well-being. I had been reading articles on the internet that resonated with me. *Time* magazine detailed how sitting was the "new cancer." Sitting in a nonergonomic chair, hunched over a computer screen for hours on end, was taking a toll on my body. The sedentary lifestyle was simple, but its effects were brutal. I could feel the aches, pains, and other symptoms of old age creeping in, prematurely aging me. If this is how I was feeling in my thirties, the future didn't seem too bright.

But I wasn't one to sit idly by. As always, my curious mind delved into health-related research topics, determined to find a way to deaccelerate the way I was aging. I knew I had to make a change, and I was willing to take action. To my surprise, an opportunity presented itself at work. The bank offered to pay for college-level courses for those who wanted to further their education. It didn't even have to be financially related, which intrigued me. I felt it was time to seize the chance to learn something new, to challenge myself beyond my comfort zone.

I had a good feeling about moving forward in a direction that emphasized physical motion. Months earlier, one of my brothers had sent me an article via email. It was a Wednesday. As usual, I'd forwarded the email to several coworkers. By the end of the day, it had spread to every employee's in-box. Most emails were silly and would lead to a chuckle or a conversation. This one was different. At least for me it was. The moment I read it, I got the feeling it had value. It was a few short paragraphs with bright drawings of fruits and vegetables. It warned against eating a banana and bread together at the same meal. The combination of fruits and refined starch would cause fermentation in the stomach. I had to look up the definition of the word *ferment*. It meant to incite trouble or cause disorder. In this context, ferment could cause discomfort and lead to more serious health issues if continued as a habit. The email suggested eating strictly fresh fruit on Friday, Saturday, and Sunday. I was anything but venturesome when it came to food. I like what I like and had been eating the same things for many years. But something kept telling me that this email was meant for me to read. More energy, clearer skin, whiter eyes, better sleep, and a boost in overall health were some of the benefits that were promised. I couldn't remember an offer sounding this good without some sort of catch. But I couldn't find one.

Unlike most of the other emails we circulated among one another, this one generated no further discussion. Not a single word from anyone. That's what I'd anticipated. It served as a social experiment. Although it guaranteed the transformation most overweight and sick people in that office needed, it required more change than they were willing to commit to. I, too, was guilty of sitting back and kicking my feet up in the comfort zone. I needed to confirm to myself that I wanted the health I spoke about. Knowing what to do and actually doing it can be worlds apart. A wise person once said, "When the student is ready, the teacher will appear." I was as ready as ever.

I decided to hit the supermarket that same day to prepare myself for the shift I knew was possible. Navel oranges, strawberries, and pineapples were the fruits I chose to eat whenever I was hungry. It was an unprecedented amount of fruit for me, as I had always viewed fruit as a sporadic snack or an appetizer before a main meal. The only time I remembered eating such copious amounts of fruit was when soccer moms would offer us orange slices after games in middle school—a distant memory. But now, fruit was my only meal, and I was amazed at how my body reacted. I visited the bathroom at least several times each day. It felt like my body was purging itself of demons. It wasn't hard to figure out why the email encouraged trying this at the end of the workweek. I got so hungry after the second day that I ate all the fruit and had to return to the market again. By the end of the third day, everything the email said would happen actually did. I'd found a reset button of sorts. I felt great. It was becoming clearer to me that what my coworkers and I had been putting in our mouths was hurting us. The article in the email was signed by Dr. Herbert Shelton, whose name I looked up on Google, leading me to discover other health pioneers: Arnold Ehret, Sylvester Graham, Isaac Jennings, and Russell Trall. This ultimately led me down a rabbit hole of articles about a system called the natural hygiene movement.

I wanted to learn more about this fruitarian lifestyle that Shelton was linked to. I kept digging for information about eating plants and came across other names, such as Dick Gregory, Dr. Sebi, and Dr. Aris LaTham. The latter had a motto that made sense to me: "It's not the food in your life, but the life in your food that nourishes." After reading dozens of articles on the internet, I found courses online. I began to envision myself as a personal trainer—a more holistic trainer than the stereotypical meathead model I had seen lurking in fitness clubs. I wanted to be on my feet, helping others overcome common health issues. Teaching proper nutrition and fitness techniques would be fun. Through my own experience, I knew that knowing what foods to eat and what foods to avoid was where most of us failed. There were so many different opinions on the subject. Charismatic characters spoke with such conviction and passion. Some had vast arrays of academic credentials but no long-term experience or true understanding of what they spoke about. To anyone unfamiliar with wellness, it was a challenge to know who or what was right. I studied the course descriptions of the University of Natural Health. The school was teaching what I needed to learn. Its philosophy was right in line with what I was already studying and implementing with degrees of success. Shelton's books were among others noted as required reading.

I began to realize that staying young and vibrant was about not only physical health but also mental and intellectual stimulation. So I enrolled in courses that piqued my interest, expanding my knowledge and feeding my passion for learning. It was a rejuvenating experience, and I could feel my mind staying sharp and agile. It was a turning point for me. I made a commitment to myself not to let a sedentary lifestyle accelerate the aging process. I incorporated regular exercise into my daily routine, made ergonomic adjustments to my work space, and prioritized mental and intellectual wellness. I was learning how to take control of my health and well-being, and the results kept improving.

Weeks later, a large box filled with thick textbooks and course folders arrived at my doorstep. Among them was a book entitled *The 80/10/10 Diet*, written by Dr. Doug Graham, which was required reading for the course. As I delved into its pages, I came across a fascinating discussion of the diets of various animals, and it struck me how each species has its own unique dietary requirements. Observing the animals around me, I couldn't help but notice that they all followed a species-specific diet, and it got me thinking about our own species. With our color vision, humans are able to discern when fruits are ripe and ready for consumption, and I personally have always been drawn to the aroma and hue of fruits like mangoes and apples. There's just nothing like the taste of a perfectly ripe fruit. Unlike other animals, I have never been tempted to pick up a dead animal on the side of the road and consume it. I didn't see sharp fangs when I opened my mouth and looked in the mirror. My teeth look like those of all of the other animals that eat vegetation.

I came upon a May 1979 article in *The New York Times* that discussed the work of Dr. Alan Walker and his associates, anthropologists at John Hopkins University. Using the most modern electronic microscopic equipment, Dr. Walker examined the wear patterns on the chewing surfaces of teeth. Boyce Rensberger, the author of the article, stated, "Preliminary studies of fossil teeth have led an anthropologist to the startling suggestion that early human ancestors were not predominantly meat eaters or even eaters of seeds, shoots, leaves or grasses, nor were they omnivorous. Instead, they appear to have subsisted chiefly on a diet of fruit." The article went on to say, "Every tooth examined from the hominids of the 12-million-year period leading up to Homo Erectus appeared to be that of a fruit-eater."

In addition to the books required for the class, I searched the internet for videos by doctors outside the curriculum. I came across a few videos with interviews of Milton Mills, M.D., an internal medicine specialist. He said some things that made me pay closer attention to the behavior of different animals in their natural habitat. He pointed out that true predators in nature always seek "ugly" foods. All of the wildlife documentaries I watched confirmed this. Nature's most skilled hunters are the wild animals that must kill to survive. They prefer prey that requires the least expenditure of energy as possible. Weak or wounded animals are their favored targets. I've always admired how calculating big cats are. As predators, they can't afford to waste all their energy without a kill. They wouldn't be able to survive if they did.

Herbivores like deer, on the other hand, look for the freshest, most "beautiful" foods. Beauty symbolizes health. I found this information relatable to me right away. There was never a time when I found myself in the produce section looking for rotten tomatoes rather than perfectly ripe ones. Carnivores have eyesight that is optimized for seeing at night and following the movement of prey. Their sense of smell is 100,000 times more powerful than mine. Lions can easily detect injured or weak prey from hundreds of yards away. These carnivorous attributes allow them to use the least amount of energy possible. I noticed that the largest land animals on this planet are herbivores. They eat plants, the source of all protein. The carnivores are always using their teeth for ripping, tearing, and cutting. My teeth couldn't do that. Mine are designed for grinding. Carnivores can swallow raw meat without chewing. Humans have to grind food by chewing in order to extract the nutrients from tissues in fruits and vegetables. I observed these phenomena in my surroundings, further confirming my beliefs about the natural world's wisdom.

The book *Topics in Dietary Fiber Research* states, "The role of dietary fiber in the preagricultural subsistence economy of early human populations strongly suggests that for over 99% of man's existence as a distinct species, his gastrointestinal tract has been exposed to the selective pressures exerted by a coarse, high-residue diet of plant tissues."

As I was learning and applying all this newfound information, I set out each day to get better without putting too much pressure on myself. Some food obsessions take longer to disappear than others. Pizza, cheesecake, sugary cereals, and ranch-flavored chips were some of the ones that lingered. A few of my taste attachments were psychological. I began to realize that I could enjoy the good memories I associated with certain foods without having to partake of them. What can I do to positively improve my health today? This was a question I began to ask myself each day. The well-being of nonhuman animals is important. But my health was the main focus. I was increasing my awareness and seeing positive changes.

As I reflect on my journey toward better health, I realize that one of the greatest obstacles I faced was leaving my comfort zone—that familiar place where progress cannot flourish. I know I'm not alone in this struggle, but I am grateful that I summoned the courage to take that initial step. Adopting a diet of minimally processed plants has had an immeasurable positive impact on my well-being. While change can be an unsettling concept for many of us, adapting to new circumstances may sound more appealing. Nonetheless, our ability to thrive in a world that is constantly evolving hinges on our willingness to cultivate a healthy lifestyle and take care of the only planet we have to call home.

> **GEMS:** In my travels across different states, countries, and continents, I've noticed that people who ate more minimally processed plants showed less facial wrinkling. Antioxidants in plants are known for decreasing oxidative stress and potential damage from the sun, improving collagen production, and strengthening DNA's ability to make repairs. All of these qualities usually result in fewer wrinkles. So far, it's worked for me.

10

FAST OR SLOW: HITTING LIFE'S RESET BUTTON

Fasting is the first principle of medicine; fast and see the strength of the spirit reveal itself.
— Rumi

During health classes I was taught that we can not live long without food. Three to six weeks without food pushes the limits of human endurance, and the time line is even shorter when it comes to water. Vital organs like the brain and heart are made up of 80 percent water. I haven't heard of anyone who could survive more than a few days without water.

I couldn't understand how people were able to live without having enough to eat or drink. I've always loved to eat. On Sunday's, the local television stations would run charity commercials that showed starving kids in Africa. The young kids were too weak to swat away the flies that landed on their drooling faces. Those haunting images left a lasting impression on me. I couldn't comprehend how their bloated bellies persisted despite their lack of nourishment. It was the sight of their protruding ribs, barely concealed by paper-thin skin, that struck me the hardest. I could only imagine the agony they must have felt. These were kids who deserved to play, laugh, and relish life, just like me. They had families who cared for them, too, but their access to the plentiful resources that surrounded them was cruelly denied to them.

It dawned on me then how fortunate I was to be born into a loving family with the means to ensure that food was always on our table. But for those less fortunate, their struggle for health and well-being was a constant battle. This realization planted the seeds for better health, propelling me into a journey of extensive research, self-discovery, and trial and error. I was determined to make the most of the abundant resources available to me, and to share my discoveries with those who needed it the most.

The devastating earthquake that shook Haiti in 2010 was a turning point in my life. Suddenly, I found myself grappling with the uncertainty of not knowing where or when my next meal would come. Food and water, once taken for granted, became precious commodities in the blink of an eye. My family and I were thrust into a crisis situation, and our survival instincts kicked in. In those harrowing moments, my mind and body kicked into overdrive, focused solely on keeping us alive. We breathed in the acrid air heavy with the stench of death, and the toll it took on our bodies and minds was palpable. We were forever marked by that harrowing experience.

In those dark days, I learned a profound lesson about the difference between hunger and appetite. Appetite, I realized, was simply a response to emotions—a way to fill a void when I was happy, sad, or bored. But true hunger, the gnawing pain that comes from prolonged lack of sustenance, was an entirely different beast. It was a primal force that gripped my gut and demanded attention.

After returning to the safety of the States, I couldn't take for granted the luxury of unlimited access to food anymore. I had tasted the desperation of true hunger, and it had awakened a hunger within me for better health and well-being. My journey to find balance had just begun. I knew that a change was required from the inside out. That's the message every cell in my body was sending me through visions in my sleep. All I kept seeing was a translucent silhouette of the digestive system in my body. Something was not right inside. I dreamed that every time I ate, the food would drop down my esophagus and come back up slowly. It was more than just a dream. When I woke, I felt the same feeling I'd envisioned. It was a seamless transition from unconscious to conscious. I began to read books and articles on the internet about fasting and how much it differed from a food addict's worst fear: starving.

An excerpt from *Staying Healthy with Nutrition: The Complete Guide to Diet and Nutritional Medicine,* by Elson M. Haas M.D., reads: "Throughout the centuries, many doctors have treated a variety of patients and maladies with fasting, acknowledging that ignorance (of how to live in accordance with nature) may be our greatest disease. Knowledge, not necessarily from books, but our inherent and experienced knowing of how to live according to the natural laws and spiritual truth, leads to the sacred wisdom of life and subsequent good health. Knowing when and how long to fast is part of this knowledge. Through fasting, we can turn our energies inward, where we can use them for healing, clarity, and change."

Those words were waiting for me to read them. When I quieted my mind and listened to the internal voice, it led me in the direction of fasting. The information I read further confirmed that I was ready to give fasting a try.

I had scoured every corner of the internet, delved into countless books, and consulted with various experts in my relentless pursuit of better health. But amid all the overwhelming information, there was one process that stood out, a proven way to extend the human life span: caloric restriction.

It was like hitting the reset button on my body, just like rebooting my computer when it wasn't working properly. By tapping into the nutritional reserves my body had stored over time, I could rejuvenate my system and get it running smoothly again. The higher the quality of those nutritional reserves, the better tools my body had to work with to make repairs. It was a primal instinct, similar to how animals in the wild instinctively fast when injured during battle. Even major religions mentioned fasting in their teachings; I remembered learning in Catholic school that Jesus had fasted for forty days and forty nights.

As I watched nature shows on television, my fascination with big cats grew. They were the epitome of strength, agility, and fearlessness. I noticed how lions in the wild would abstain from food when injured, conserving their energy for healing rather than digestion. It was a natural instinct, and I couldn't help but wonder if fasting could be the simplest and most natural method of detoxifying my body.

The commercials on television showing starving children broke my heart. I learned that starvation occurred when nutritional reserves were completely depleted and vital tissues were broken down just to sustain life. It was a harsh reality that underscored the importance of proper nutrition and the significance of fasting as a method to reset and optimize our bodies.

With each new discovery, I was driven to know more. The concept of fasting intrigued me, and I was eager to explore this ancient practice that seemed to hold the key to unlocking better health. I was determined to uncover the truth.

Fasting was so much more than just abstaining from food. It was a way of giving my body the rest it desperately needed, and there were different methods to achieve that. I was intrigued by the concept of dry fasting—going without food or water—and decided to give it a shot. I'll admit, I wasn't sure how far I'd get, but I was determined to try. The first twenty-four hours were tough. The urge to eat constantly nagged at me, and I found myself checking the time every other hour, hoping that time would somehow pass more quickly. I searched the internet for articles on fasting to keep my mind occupied until I eventually drifted off to sleep. I soon realized that the key was to gain control over my thoughts. Once I had my mind on board, my body put up less resistance. It was a fascinating realization—the power of the mind over the body in overcoming the challenges of fasting.

I was determined to explore different methods of fasting, and one that caught my attention was juice fasting—a period of consuming only fruit or vegetable juice. I felt confident I could handle it, as the juice would still provide essential nutrients my body absorbs like vitamins, minerals, glucose, and water, allowing me to continue most of my normal activities. Juicing removes fiber that passes through my digestive tract undigested. With less fiber, uptake of some nutrients would slow while glucose absorption would quicken. I was interested in experimenting with active rest while still nourishing my body.

Then there was water fasting, which seemed to be more challenging. I wasn't a fan of drinking plain water unless I was incredibly thirsty—it lacked taste and aroma. But I knew it was a powerful approach to fasting, as distilled water is used in medical, dental, and chemical laboratories for sanitation purposes. Even doctors use it in operating rooms to clean wounds and prevent infections. I was convinced that it could have the same cleansing effect on my insides.

I decided to start my water fast on a Thursday night, as it wouldn't interfere with my work schedule. I stocked up on several gallons of distilled water from the store and set a goal of completing seventy-two hours without any other form of nourishment. It was a bold undertaking, but I was up for the challenge. I knew it wouldn't be easy, but I was willing to push through, knowing that come Monday, I would resume eating again. The anticipation of embarking on this journey filled me with a sense of excitement and determination.

As I savored my last meal on Thursday around 7:00 P.M., I knew that the next few days would be a test of my resolve. I wanted to start my fast while I slept, so I could wake up with several hours already under my belt. The first day, Friday, surprisingly went by smoothly. I woke up, drank a couple of glasses of water, and headed to work at the bank. Despite my usual routine of taking a lunch break between 1:00 and 2:00 P.M., I didn't feel any signs of hunger. It was strange to break away from my usual pattern, especially since I was a regular at the sandwich shop next door. The overpowering smell of chemicals from the bread they used was always noticeable, and some of my coworkers had even commented on how I smelled like bread after lunch. But now, with my senses heightened during the fast, I could smell the lingering scent of bread on my colleagues when they returned from lunch. It was a realization that caught me off guard.

Throughout the day, I found myself instinctively checking the clock at the times when I would normally eat. It was a habit that was deeply ingrained in my daily routine, and now it was a reminder of the challenge I had taken on. Despite the moments of temptation and the awareness of the passing time, I remained committed to my fast, knowing that it was a step toward better health and self-discovery. The sense of discipline and control that I gained from this experience was empowering, and I was eager to see how the rest of the fast would unfold.

The second day was tougher. The good thing was, I didn't have to go to work. The emotional roller coaster of deep detox is a wild ride. It was also somewhat comforting to know that the symptoms I was experiencing resulted from normal resistance by the mind. Going without food made me realize something. Eating was a convenient distraction. It wasn't long before old thoughts returned: Maybe this isn't the best time to try this. Twenty-four hours without food was great; let's stop now and try again some other time.

Why am I doing this again? The detox demons were trying to talk me out of completing this task. My energy felt depleted—nowhere near as high as the day before. The irritability I'd read about tried to creep into my conscience. I kept drinking water anytime I felt hungry. Food is like a drug. It was time to slow down and address the fasting symptoms that my research said would be knocking. What began as a rest for my digestive system also became a hiatus from mental toxins, as well. I limited my consumption of negative media. Before the fast, I didn't pay much attention to all the food advertising that surrounded me. I knew it was there, but I didn't understand how prevalent it really was. Television, radio in the car, billboards on buses and benches, intrusive internet ads, etc., were always promoting unhealthy food. The media programming was especially true in lower-income neighborhoods. I couldn't pass by any fast-food restaurant without catching a whiff of the toxic oils and dead animals that were cooking inside.

The power of my mind to shape my perception of health, whether positively or negatively, was a strength that I had underestimated. By the time the third day of my fast arrived, I had surpassed the initial pangs of hunger. I had learned that true hunger originated from the mouth area, not the rumbling sensations in the stomach that I had always associated with it. My breathing had slowed down, each breath became deliberate and intentional. With fewer internal distractions, I found myself more attuned to my surroundings. I could hear the ticking of the pendulum clock that had hung on the wall for years. My heartbeat seemed stronger, or perhaps I was just more aware of its steady rhythm. I noticed streaks on glass surfaces in my vicinity, and when I looked into a mirror to check my eyes, I noticed that they were whiter than before. The songs of the birds outside were distinctly clear, and I found myself forming authentic connections with the people I interacted with as I slowed down each interaction and savored the present moment, which would typically fly by in my mind.

Although my legs felt like rubber pegs, I immersed myself in reading, finding that my concentration was sharper. I only stood up when I needed to use the bathroom, as my frequent urination persisted due to the gallon of water I was drinking daily. When I focused my attention on a task, the hunger spells seemed to diminish.

Finally, the time came to break my fast, and I started with a small bowl of diced watermelon that I had prepared the night before. It tasted like the most delicious fruit I had ever had. My taste buds were heightened and extra sensitive, and each mouthful of the juicy watermelon exploded with sweet flavor, quenching my thirst and satisfying my senses. The density of flavor in each bite was exactly what my body needed after the fast, and it was a moment of pure appreciation for the simple pleasure of food.

If only I'd known earlier. The seasonal colds, flus, asthma attacks, mucus congestion episodes, constipation, hemorrhoids, digestive dramas, headaches, and other issues could have been properly addressed by letting my body solve the problem on its own.

Since then, I've gone on to completing a seven-day water fast. I've also done twenty-one-day juice and smoothie fasts. The juices are made at low speeds with the fiber removed. The smoothies are blended at high speeds with added water while keeping the fiber. I found both to be effective in giving my digestive organs a rest while promoting healing and recovery. The end results have always been clearer skin, improved digestion, heightened awareness, fat loss, elimination of symptoms, and increased energy, among other positive outcomes.

> **GEMS:** Fasting has been a reliable tool of transformation for me. It's elongated fasting that I've found effective on an almost daily basis. Fourteen to sixteen hours without eating has been great for allowing my internal organs to rest and repair during the catabolic metabolic cycle. A window of eight hours to eat has worked well to satisfy me without

binging. Juice fasts are awesome for those days I'm looking to rest internally while continuing to work. Water fasts are life-changing as well, but I wouldn't recommend they be done unsupervised, especially by those who are not in great health or have no previous fasting experience.

11

TOOTHACHE TO TRIUMPH: HEALING FROM WITHIN, ONE BITE AT A TIME

Love conquers all things except poverty and toothache.
— *Mae West*

Somewhere in school I was taught that whenever you lost a tooth as a child, the tooth fairy would visit you while you slept. You'd wake up with money underneath your pillow and comfort in knowing that teeth grow back eventually. I wanted to lose as many teeth as possible. At the time, it seemed like a profitable practice. As I matured, I realized we didn't have an endless supply of backup teeth.

One afternoon, upon returning home from a long work shift at a bank, excruciating pain boomeranged from my mouth to my brain. It felt like an evil spirit was stomping through my brain and stabbing my gums and teeth with razor-sharp pins and needles. I called the nearest dentist's office and mumbled, "I have an emergency. A major one. I need to see a dentist as soon as possible!"

After I further explained my pain, the receptionist told me the dentist was booked for the day. The earliest-possible appointment wasn't until the next day. As disheartened as I was, I didn't have much of a choice. I took some over-the-counter chemicals to try to numb the pain.

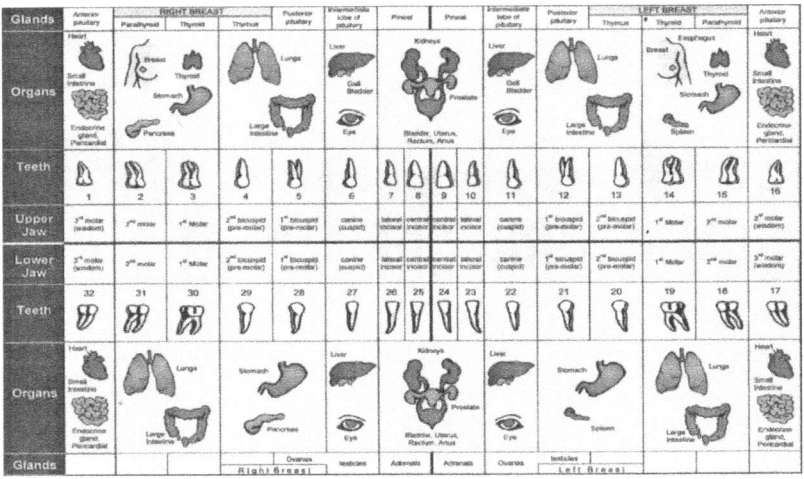

Tooth/Organ Relationship Chart

Tossing and turning throughout the night, I kept asking myself where this discomfort was coming from. My previous dentist, a dental student at Stony Brook University, did warn me of possible dental problems in the future. He also told me that I unknowingly grind my teeth at night, perhaps due to anxiety and stress. That was several years earlier. Yes, it had been a while. Like most people, I had always had jitters about visiting the dentist. I remembered all the cavities and the painful procedures to drill and fill them in. The sound of the drill is traumatic at best. The last thing I looked forward to was sitting in the dentist's chair, but I had to do something.

The next day, the dentist's X-ray revealed that one of my wisdom teeth was indeed the root of the problem (sorry, that was tasteless). Unfortunately, that wasn't the only issue I was dealing with. More tests showed that I had periodontal disease, a form of chronic, low-grade inflammation. My wisdom teeth were impacted, and my gums were infected and extremely sensitive to the touch. The flossing the dentist did right then and there led to bleeding. I was never a proponent of flossing. It was tedious and always hurt. My periodontitis was so advanced, the dentist said it would require pocket-reduction surgery. He detailed a multistep process that would require multiple cleaning visits.

"If I remove the wisdom tooth, I have to warn you of the possible complications."

"You mean to tell me that I could potentially still have problems after the surgery?"

"Yes, let me show you. You see this tooth right here?" he asked, pointing to the X-ray.

"I see it."

"It's sitting right on top of the fifth cranial nerve, also called the trigeminal nerve."

"That doesn't sound good."

"Most wisdom teeth come in around twenty-five; you're almost forty."

"Thanks for reminding me," I said, half-joking.

"The teeth are so impacted way in the back. If we perform the surgery, there is a real risk of damaging the nerve."

"If the nerve is damaged, can it heal?"

"That depends on how severe the damage is. Minor damage can heal in a few weeks or months. Major damage can be permanent."

Ever since my twenties, I'd ignored the dentist's recommendations of checkups every six months. Having to return again before the end of the month didn't excite me. The idea of possible permanent damage had me worried. I had a flashback of squirming, flinching, bleeding, and shedding tears while clutching the armrest of the dentist's chair during the last cleaning. That could've been just a dream. But it was clear why I didn't like going to the dentist.

I tried to get a clear answer before I left.

So, what is the cause of the periodontal disease?"

"It's usually a result of poor brushing and flossing, especially not brushing after each meal. These habits allowed the plaque to build up and harden over time."

Although I hadn't flossed in years, I wasn't satisfied with that answer.

I went home and gave the situation deep thought. I came across an article titled "Diet Related to Killer Diseases: Hearings Before the Select Committee." It read: "It is now conclusively proven by numerous independent studies (Cleveland Clinic, University of Wisconsin, Brigham Young University, etc.) that the high phosphorus content of meat results in loss of calcium from the bones."

I had been devouring internet health articles for months. "Periodontal Disease and Diabetes—A Two Way Street Dual Highway?" by Dr. J. Deshmukh and others mentioned the difficulty people with periodontal disease had in controlling their blood-sugar levels. Discovering that most sufferers of diabetes also had periodontal disease gave me additional cause for concern. I had relatives who had acquired type 2 diabetes. It was time for me to apply what I was learning and commit to a lifestyle change.

The fruit fast I'd done months before gave me great results. It even helped me get rid of the sporadic stomach pains I had been experiencing. I already knew what was needed to manifest the positive changes I was looking for. The books I had been reading and the way I felt after just three days eating minimally processed plant foods made so much sense. My daily eating habits were taking a toll on my teeth. Especially, the cooked foods I was eating every day. It was either I execute this metamorphosis in my mind or commit to the surgery. Refined grains, animal products, and heavily processed foods were what led to the buildup of plaque on my gums and teeth. The statistics from the American College of Prosthodontists website stated that "more than 36 million Americans do not have any teeth, and 120 million people in the U.S. are missing at least one tooth." When I looked at my surroundings at work, the stores I shopped at, family, etc., these numbers matched up. Bad teeth can make a person look and feel decades older. I didn't know many people over the age of fifty who had their real teeth. I would notice popular actors and singers on television and in magazines. Some of them were missing teeth. They must have practiced poor dental hygiene, like I did. All of a sudden, they would make public appearances with bright, pearly white teeth. For celebrities, getting veneers was the popular thing to do. A dentist would place a certain material over the teeth and make them appear shiny. Some people consider a set of veneers to be a symbol of wealth and prestige. They looked like big piano keys in a person's mouth.

I later learned that each tooth in my mouth is related to an organ in the body. By closely observing my teeth, I could discern the level of health in the corresponding organ. Meridian networks interconnect certain organs to specific teeth using a number system. Each tooth is given a number from 1 to 32. Two of the teeth I felt pain in were teeth 28 and 29. Tooth 29, also known as the second bicuspid (premolar), is connected to the stomach. I had been experiencing bloating, acid reflux, and fatigue. Tooth 28, also known as the first bicuspid (premolar), is connected to the pancreas. One potential consequence of a weak pancreas is diabetes. Type 2 diabetes is prevalent on my maternal side of the family. Using a tooth/organ relationship chart, I could determine how each organ in my mouth affected a given tooth. Discomfort in the affected areas went away once I made the appropriate dietary changes.

As jacked up as they were, I liked my teeth and I didn't have any money for veneers. Besides, veneers might improve the aesthetics but wouldn't address the true cause of the problem. I took the chemical pills the dentist prescribed and drove to the nearest grocery store to buy as many fruits and vegetables as my budget would allow. I also picked up toothpaste that didn't contain fluoride. Although I wasn't swallowing fluoride, I read some of the hundreds of animal and human studies done on it. They proved that it was a neurotoxin, which meant it was destructive to nerve tissue. Some dentists said it wasn't harmful in small amounts. But I read a World Health Organization statistic that stated over 95 percent of European countries didn't fluorinate their water supply and dental health wasn't negatively affected. A tube of non-fluoride toothpaste cost three dollars more than I was used to paying, but I figured it was worth a shot. I drank only water before going to sleep. The next morning, I woke up and stared at a photocopy of the X-ray of my infected teeth taped to my bedroom door. I decided that I would eat only minimally processed plants. Yes, a man who had eaten cooked food for over three decades would now attempt to eat strictly fruits, vegetables, nuts, seeds, and a variety of sprouts that were cooked solely by the sun.

No more rice or pasta. Gone were the breads and pastries. Oatmeal was off the table. Cheese, eggs, milk, and yogurt were now in my rearview mirror. There was no looking back to chicken, fish, or dead animal flesh of any kind. How could I expect to gain life energy from the dead corpses rotting in my intestines? If I wanted to live pain-free, then it only made sense that I consume healthy foods. I had to at least give it a try. I read articles about the importance of eating locally grown produce. I would ask the grocer questions about the farming practices where the produce was grown. The local organic farmers told me that they didn't use conventional chemical pesticides. They used pesticides derived from plant extracts, pheromones, and other naturally occurring substances that disrupt the lifecycles of pests. There were many benefits to eating seasonal foods. Food grown only a few miles away was fresher and had better taste. Since some of the nutrients can be lost just a day after the produce is picked, local foods were healthier. It was autumn in New York, so apples and pears were in season. My first meal, though, consisted of citrus fruits: three oranges, a grapefruit, and pineapple slices. These are known as acidic fruits. I read that they became alkaline once the body assimilated them. The nutrients my body was able to use was what truly mattered. I ate an assortment of fruits and vegetables three to four times a day. This went on every day for about three months. A decade earlier, I had gone on a meat-free, junk food diet, but what I was doing now was different. This was my introduction to a lifestyle of unfamiliar plant foods while excluding everything else. It was one of the most challenging things I had ever done. At times it felt like I was living on a deserted island. I didn't know anyone personally who even thought about trying this with me. Growing up as an only child really played to my advantage. Being comfortably alone with my thoughts made it easier to focus, unlearn years of misinformation, and apply the new information I was learning. I was able to block out the usual triggers that were all around me—mainly because I was teaching myself to identify familiar smells and place them in simple categories. I associated the smell of dead animals with death and dis-ease. I realized that what made meatballs smell so good was the seasoning herbs, spices, and tomatoes. Remove plants from the recipe and the meat wouldn't smell appetizing. Fresh produce was filled with water, nutrients, and stored sunlight energy. I associated these ingredients with health and wellness.

Three months later, I returned to see the dentist. Although I had never been rotund, I kept a consistent fitness routine and showed up twenty-five pounds lighter. The discomfort in my mouth was completely gone. This was the first time that I had ever been excited to see a dentist. Days earlier, I was using my front teeth to bite into crunchy apples. I felt no pain. I could feel with my tongue that the thick layer of plaque on my teeth had decreased. I sat in the dentist's chair to have more X-rays taken. I waited for the results. The dentist entered the room holding a manila envelope, a perplexed look on his face.

"I don't know what you've been doing, but keep doing it. Most of the plaque that showed during your last visit is gone," he said, showing me the new X-rays.

"I've made a few changes to my eating habits. I'm glad they're paying off," I replied.

"We'll just complete a normal cleaning today."

I was brushing my teeth twice a day, just like I always had. I flossed maybe once during those three months (maybe not the healthiest approach, but I'm still a work in progress). The holistic nutrition information I was reading and applying to my diet was working to my advantage. The animal meat, grains, and other overly processed foods I had eaten in the past were acid-forming. They created excessive amounts of acid and phosphorus in my bloodstream. This led to mineral imbalances. My body responded to the imbalances by leeching calcium from my bones and teeth to neutralize the excess acid. This explained the reason for my loss of enamel, cavities, and tooth erosion throughout the years. The live plants, on the other hand, provided the right balance of calcium, phosphorus, and various other minerals. Although my teeth remained impacted, I was able to prevent further damage. Unlike all of the soft, sticky cooked food I used to eat, fresh salads required a lot more chewing before swallowing. I wouldn't advise trying to eat an unprocessed, leafy salad without taking the time to chew thoroughly. In order to keep from choking, I had to turn each mouthful to soft mush. Eating lots of green leafy vegetables is great oral exercise. My jaw muscles were sore for days after eating a large bowl. An example of large for me would be about twelve cups of uncooked kale. Salad just wasn't something I was used to eating in bulk. I soon made it a point to eat at least one large salad daily. Carnivores need bones for calcium and jaw exercise. I need leafy greens for calcium and to work my face, neck, and jaw muscles.

When speaking to those in the dental office, I was not specific about the alterations I had made to my diet. The dentist didn't show any curiosity to know more. That was disappointing. Just three months earlier, my mouth had been a disaster zone. How many of his patients had ever done what I just had? Zero would be a safe bet. This was Long Island, New York. I grew up here, and knew the food culture as well as anybody. I smiled and left the office, feeling like the wealthiest man in the world. I learned valuable lessons at the dentist's office that day. Dentists are well educated. Their degrees cost what most people around the world would consider a small fortune. The hours of clinical study and research require discipline, sacrifice, and commitment. With all of that said, their education is limited. It does not teach them the common causes of the dental deterioration issues that oral care professionals see on a daily basis. Food choices. Sure, most of us know that refined sugars and junk foods are not healthy. I now understand that it's much deeper than that. *Junk food* was both an obvious and vague term to me. It was time to be specific. I kept a daily journal of everything I ate and drank for months. I documented how they made me feel afterward. The chemical reactions that occur in my body when I eat minimally processed plants are favorable. The feedback is not as agreeable when I eat anything else—especially when consumed for prolonged periods of time. That helped me make the distinction between what was junk and what was healthy. It felt good to apply better information. The learning process continues to have a positive impact on my quality of life.

> **GEMS:** Eating a large, uncooked leafy green salad every day requires more time, patience, and jaw muscle activity than a plate of cooked food. It's also one of the most effective ways to avoid a double chin or buffalo hump on the back of the neck as we age.

12

REDEMPTION IN RED: A BATTLE AGAINST EYE AGONY

When I look into the future, it's so bright it burns my eyes.
— *Oprah Winfrey*

It was a frigid February day on Long Island, New York, and I was desperate for warmth. The dirty snow and icy streets only added to my desire to escape. So I decided to use my ten days of vacation time from work to visit my parents in sunny Florida. However, for weeks prior, I had been dealing with a bothersome sensation in my left eye. It felt like there were tiny grains of sand moving around beneath my eyelid, causing discomfort and strain whenever I looked up at the sky. Sometimes it was a minor annoyance, while other times it was so severe that it would stop me in my tracks. I noticed a filmy discharge and attempted to alleviate the blurry vision by rubbing my eyes or using over-the-counter eyedrops. But it was clear that something more serious was going on.

Despite some turbulence during the flight, I arrived at my parents' house without any major issues. They were overjoyed to see me, and I was relieved to see that they were doing well. However, I quickly excused myself, claiming that I needed rest from the long flight, when in reality, it was my troublesome eye that was bothering me. I couldn't pinpoint the exact cause—it could have been the change in altitude during the flight or the sudden increase in temperature upon arriving in Florida, where it was over eighty degrees, with high humidity. The pesky insects with their stingers didn't help, either. No matter what I tried, my vision remained blurry, and rubbing my eyes only seemed to make it worse. Closing my eyes provided temporary relief, but upon opening them, it felt like there was a persistent film of dust covering my lens. I attempted to take a nap, hoping that I would wake up with improved vision, but unfortunately, it didn't happen. My frustration grew, and I was losing patience quickly. How could I possibly enjoy the rest of my visit with this nagging issue persisting?

I went into the bathroom and examined my eye in the mirror. It was bloodshot and irritated from all the rubbing. I decided to wash my hands thoroughly with soap and warm water for a minute before attempting to address the issue. With my eyes tightly closed, I used my left index finger to carefully touch my eyelid, and I could feel something between my eyeball and eyelid. An idea struck me. I had dealt with a similar situation before when the end of a drawstring on my boxer briefs would get lost in the waistband, and I would have to feel around, squeeze, and pull it toward the drawstring hole to retrieve it. That's exactly what I needed to do with whatever was stuck in my eyelid.

With gentle movements, I massaged the bump downward towards my eyelash, and I could feel it moving. I wiped away the tears that followed with a paper towel. After several minutes of this careful maneuvering, I blinked rapidly and finally opened my eyes. To my amazement, there was a thin white film covering my eye horizontally from one corner to the other. It was the cause of weeks of discomfort, and my eye was now even redder from all the rubbing.

I decided to rest my eye and took another one-hour nap, all the while contemplating how I was going to resolve this issue. I knew I had to pull the stringlike object out from under my eyelid, but this time, there was no room for error. Unlike a pair of boxer shorts that could be easily replaced, I only had one left eye, and to me, it was priceless.

I opened my eyes and went to the bathroom mirror. My vision was turbid, but I could still see the filmy substance. Maybe I could carefully grab it with tweezers dipped in alcohol? No, that was too risky. I had about two millimeters of nail growth on my index finger and thumb. Maybe I could reach in and grab it that way. Standing in front of the mirror over the sink, I turned on the faucet until the water was lukewarm. I splashed water into my eye. Maybe I could flush this thing out with water. That didn't work. Next, I filled up a six-inch-deep basin, set it over the sink, and dipped my face in the water. I opened and closed my eyes, hoping to stimulate the film to move. That didn't work, either. I stood up and faced the mirror. I tried to hold my left eye open with my left hand while reaching in to grab the film with my right. Every time I tried to dip my fingernails toward my left eye, I'd instinctively blink. I started to gently feel for the film by placing my finger on my eyelid. I applied light pressure when I felt it and pushed it down. The goal was to push it toward my nose so I could grab it when it reached the corner. It was working. I felt it move. The more it moved, the more my eye began to tear. I looked in the mirror and saw a piece right where I thought I had the best chance to grab it. With my index finger and thumb, I grabbed it and pulled slowly. It was moving. I was carefully pulling this long, stringy white substance out of my eye. It felt better the more of it that came out. It sort of looked like a spider's web. I held it up to the light with both hands in triumph! I couldn't believe what I had just done. I sat down and kept my eyes closed for several minutes, with a tissue to absorb the tears.

I was finally able to open and close my eyes without restriction. I never wanted to have to do that again. It was risky. I had been taking my ability to see clearly for granted. Now I wanted to know what that was and how it had gotten there? The white film was the cause for my grainy vision, but what had caused the film to form in my eye? My relationships were healthy and I didn't think I was dealing with any more stress than the average adult. Was this a symptom of poor balance between life at work and life outside work?

After some research, I came to a conclusion. My internet searches consistently pointed toward calcium. Knowing that type 2 diabetes was prevalent on my maternal side of the family, I stumbled upon articles written by holistic doctors that suggested the cause of this condition was excess fat, particularly saturated fat. Saturated fat blocks the insulin hormone from allowing blood sugar to enter muscle and liver cells, causing sugar to accumulate outside the cells and resulting in high blood sugar. But how did this relate to calcium? Well, the concentrated protein foods I consumed, such as large amounts of chicken and fish daily, also contained high amounts of saturated fats. This excess protein increased the acidity levels in my blood, leading to an imbalanced alkaline-acid ratio, which could be dangerous. In response, my body searched for alkaline minerals to buffer the acid, and calcium in my skeletal system was the number-one alkaline store. A blood pH under 7.35 indicated high acidity, which could even result in death. Therefore, to keep me alive, my body was stripping calcium from my bones and teeth to neutralize the acid. Aging is accelerated when calcium is transferred from bones to the body's soft tissues. During this transfer, calcium fragments may have been floating around in my bloodstream. Cataracts are a common complication of type 2 diabetes, and my mom had once had cataracts in both eyes and elected to have them surgically removed. I did some simple math and concluded that due to my genetic predisposition, the white stringy substance in my left eye had to have been calcium. Cataracts is an eye condition commonly associated with elderly people, and it usually takes years for calcium to build up, calcify, and cloud a person's vision. Instead of seeing a doctor, who would have most likely prescribed experimental chemicals to temporarily relieve the symptoms, I decided to seek answers. Although I didn't completely understand what was happening, I had enough presence of mind to know that I needed to change my habits.

I was continuing to explore how interconnected everything truly is. Although I was experiencing dis-ease in my left eye, I knew that the underlying cause must be affecting my entire being. This was a serious warning sign that could not be ignored. In a weird way, I was in a great position. If what I was reading was true, then I had the power not only to prevent this from happening to me again but to help many others do the same.

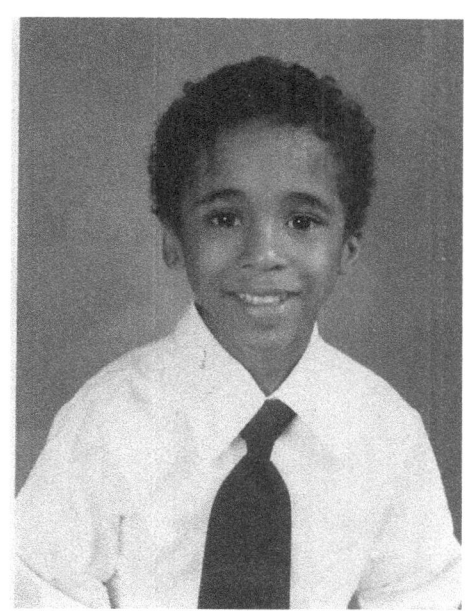

Hey young world

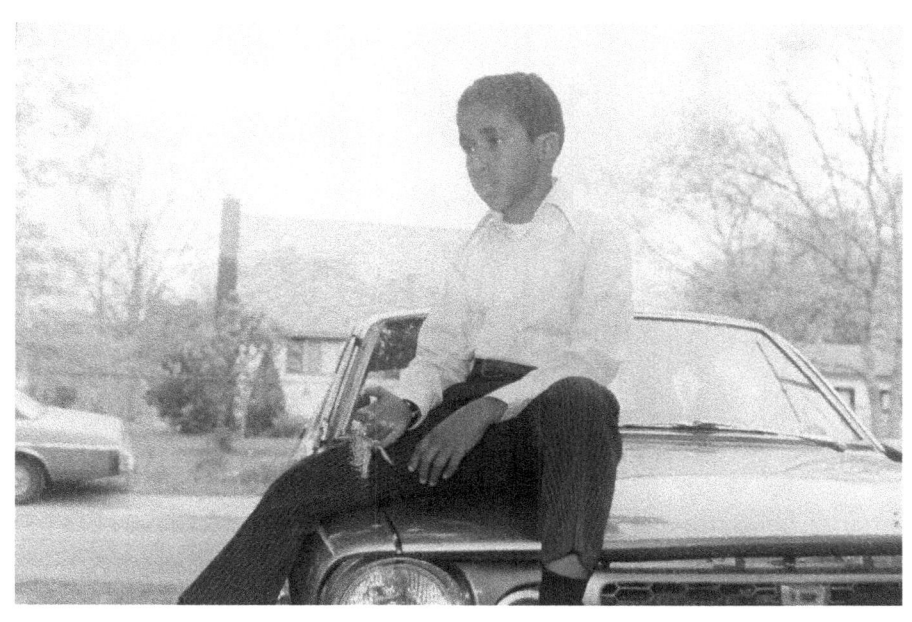

One of my first visits to Long Island from Brooklyn

WILL LOISEAU

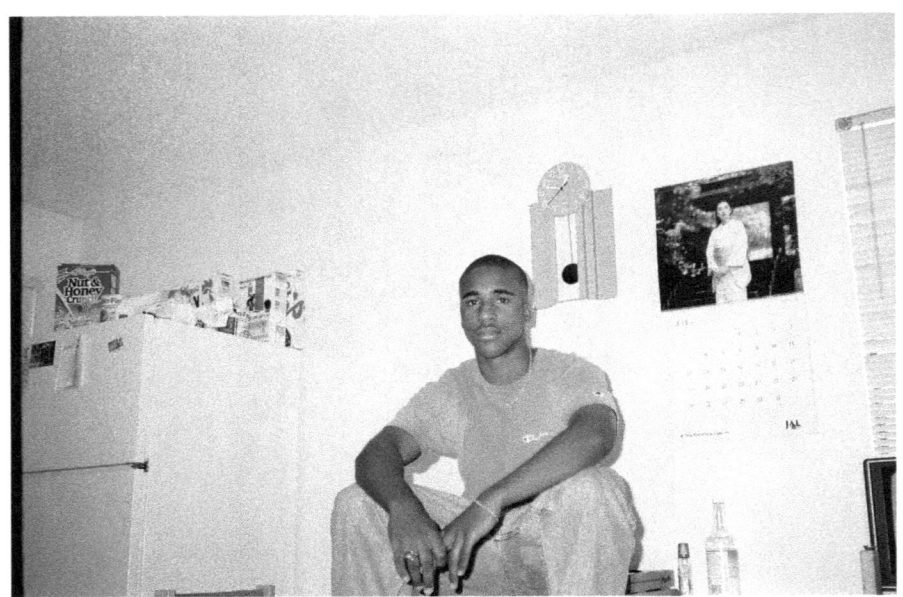

Freshman year at FIU right before Hurricane Andrew

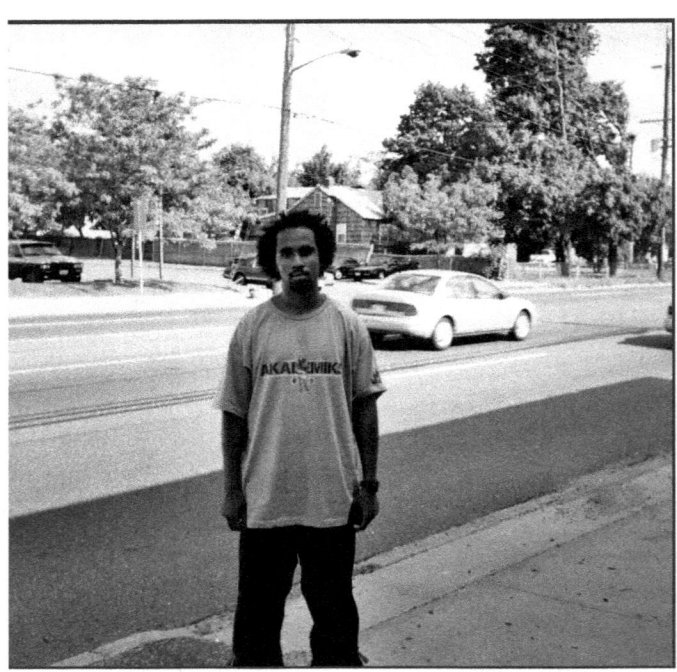

The person I had become in AZ was not the person I wanted to be on LI

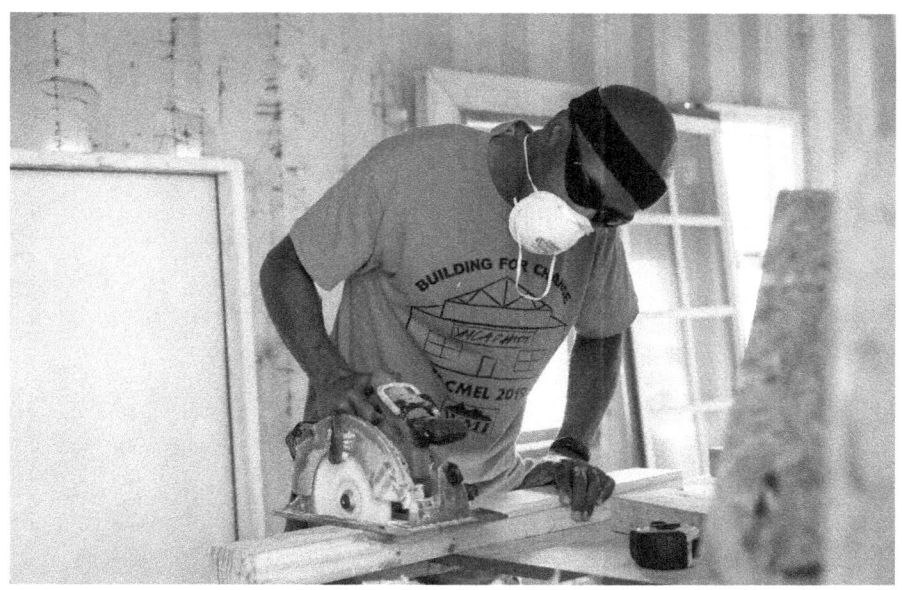

Guiding a track saw on cutting table for container project - Jacmel Haiti - Photo Credit - Madison Fender

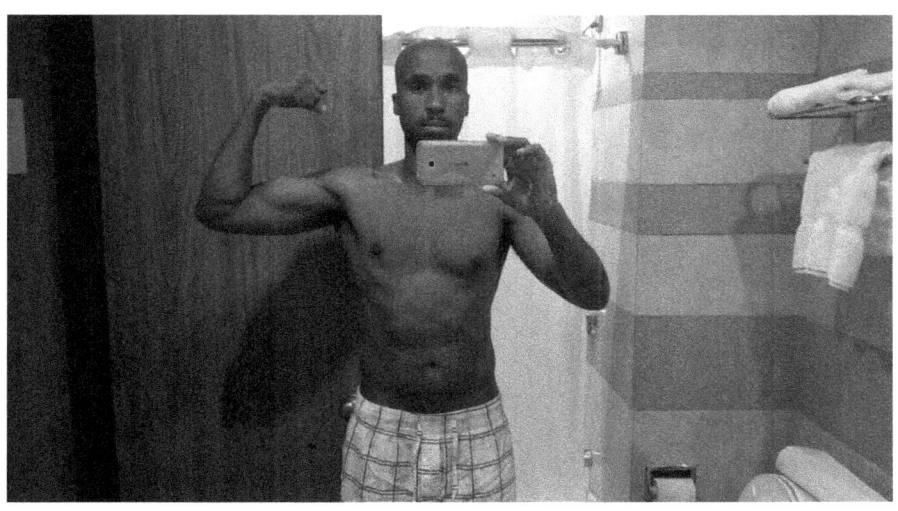

During the community center project in Haiti_ I developed confidence in maintaining a healthy lifestyle while traveling.

WILL LOISEAU

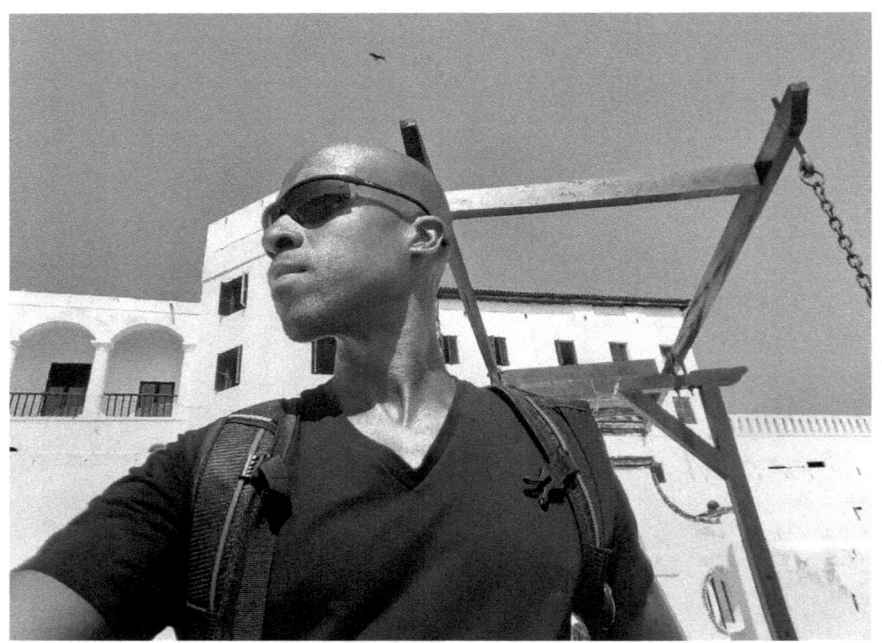

In Ghana at the Elmina Castle

13

EMBRACING THE POWER OF SELF-DISCOVERY

When you own your breath, nobody can steal your peace.
— *Anonymous*

Happiness is defined by *Merriam-Webster's* as "a state of well-being and contentment." Throughout my adult life, I've been intrigued with meeting people I never met before. Some would come up to me and say similar things. They would ask me if I was sad or upset at something. At times, this happened without fail, no matter where I went. A part of me would feel like telling them to mind their business and keep moving. If I didn't appreciate their energy, I actually did do that. I wouldn't approach someone to ask him why he talked so much. To me, that would seem strange. I was not antisocial. Reserved and quiet? Yes, that's how I tend to operate. I was a guarded individual. As an only child, I learned that the person I'd most be able to rely on was me. Although, my mother told me to trust no one, I was smart enough to know that not everyone was intentionally out to get me. Sometimes, those with the best intentions may not be in position to look out for your best interests. Other times, they may think they are helping you when actually they are hurting you. Reading world history gave me awareness of the actions people tend to echo. I gained a healthy skepticism of people who didn't look like me. I understood that history doesn't repeat itself. People repeat history. I guarded the door that could lead to my being treated unjustly. If it was someone who did look like me, my presence could trigger self-hate, a lingering effect of historical trauma. At any time, someone's reflection in the mirror can be a chilling reminder of the deep scars left by historical events. Either way, I had to be prepared to defend myself against destructive behavior people directed toward themselves or toward me.

Growing up in New York, even if it was the suburbs of Long Island, required the development of thick skin to survive.

Happiness doesn't look or feel the same for everyone. A face with a smile may not always equal a happy person. A face without one doesn't necessarily indicate sadness. Sometimes, a smile is a mask to conceal pain. At times, a neutral expression is a sign of content. Happiness for me is peace of mind. Freedom from unnecessary distractions, flexibility, and control of time brings me joy. It's helping others and knowing that I am able to contribute to something that will outlast my physical existence. Happiness is gratitude and the ability to share the gifts that the universe has given me. It's also continuously figuring out ways to utilize these gifts most effectively.

I yearned for more than mere survival in this world. To truly thrive was my ultimate goal, and I knew that I needed to make changes in my life to achieve it. Sometimes, I would take a moment to write down a list of things that brought me joy, and then I would ponder how many of those things I actually did while I was busy earning a living. The sad truth was that I had been neglecting my own happiness for far too long.

I started to pay closer attention to how I felt during certain activities. Did they bring me joy, contentment, or unhappiness? I made mental notes of my reactions and began to categorize them accordingly. The ultimate aim was to move away from the things that no longer served me, that no longer brought me the fulfillment I craved.

I had heard stories of wealthy businessmen who, despite their fortunes, still felt unfulfilled and ultimately took their own lives. Money couldn't buy them happiness or fill the void in their hearts. On the other hand, there were those who confidently charged exorbitant fees for their services, knowing full well that their time was their most valuable resource. These people had achieved something I wanted— a sense of purpose and fulfillment.

For a while, I struggled with the notion that sacrificing my precious time for things that did not bring me joy was simply a fact of life. Believing that one's self-worth is directly tied to productivity contributes to depressive thoughts. I had been mentally conditioned to believe that the reward system of our society demanded that I grin and bear it. But eventually, I realized that my time was too valuable to spend doing things that didn't truly matter to me.

The ability to master my emotions is essential for a happy life. Walking the fine line between empathizing with others but not getting lost in their feelings has been a skill I learned through my relationships with women. Those moments remain etched in my mind, as they taught me how to navigate the delicate balance between empathy and self-preservation. I learned the hard way that absorbing another person's emotional baggage can leave you feeling drained and disconnected from yourself. But that doesn't mean I shy away from empathy altogether. There are times when it's crucial to extend compassion to others. However, I've learned not to sacrifice my identity and beliefs in the process. When I'm content with who I am and the space I'm in, it's easier to invite someone else into that personal space without losing myself in the process. Taking breaks from a relationship has proved to be just as important as spending time together. It allows me to remain true to my core values without compromising for the sake of the other person.

As a younger adult, I was plagued by an insidious self-consciousness that shadowed me wherever I went. I couldn't shake the nagging feeling that, whenever I was alone in public, people would assume I was lonely. The fear of being judged by others was suffocating, and it prevented me from fully embracing my own natural inclinations.

But as I delved deeper into my own self-discovery, I realized that this fear was nothing more than a symptom of the contagious sheep mentality that seems to infect so many people. Everywhere I looked, I saw individuals struggling with their own insecurities, all the while trying to mask them with forced smiles and hollow laughter. It was only when I learned to accept myself that I was able to break free from the shackles of society's expectations. I realized that solitude was not a curse, but a gift. It allowed me to explore my own thoughts and emotions without the interference of external influences. Of course, there were moments when my internal struggles became uncomfortable, but I knew that this was a necessary part of the journey toward self-discovery.

I watched as so many of my peers settled for relationships that were less than ideal simply because they were afraid of being alone. They lived in expensive cities, crowded apartments, and shared spaces just to make ends meet. But I knew that I couldn't follow in their footsteps. I didn't want to sacrifice who I was in order to fit in a situation that wouldn't benefit me. I needed to get comfortable with myself first before I could even think about building meaningful relationships with others.

For me, happiness is a part of my journey. I see it like any skill that requires practice. It's not something that comes naturally to everyone. It's the special moments that require us to be present and cherish the elements that go into creating a joyous atmosphere. The recipe for happiness begins in the mind and it takes time and effort to perfect it.

Five years after the devastating earthquake in Haiti, something felt off in my life. Part of it was survivor's guilt, but there was something more. I spent countless nights dreaming about being back there. I wasn't grieving; I was having the time of my life in those dreams. Serving others has always given me a sense of purpose, and I knew that's what I needed.

That summer, I met an architect who was heading to Haiti to work on a project with the YMCA. He showed me pictures of completed projects in various cities, and I was beyond excited. My brother had told me that what I was searching for was also searching for me, and it seemed like fate. That fall, I joined a group of more than a dozen people to construct a community center out of shipping containers. It was the toughest work I had ever done. I had no previous construction experience, and the heat was nearly unbearable. We worked long hours, lifting, drilling, measuring, cutting, and cleaning. The kids from the neighborhood passed by every day on their way home from school, and the elders watched us work with admiration. We were using our abilities to help rebuild a country that had been devastated by an earthquake. It was a priceless feeling.

Giving is a natural human behavior, but it seems to be becoming a lost art. While it may not be as celebrated as receiving, it's much more gratifying. Seeing the excitement and joy on the faces of the people who would benefit from our work made it all worth it. That experience taught me that accepting my strengths and challenges will lead to a happier life.

What impressed me the most was the strength of the people. Despite not having any material wealth, their perspectives were unique. They were happy just to open their eyes in the morning, to walk and feel the sun's rays, to spend time with loved ones, and to have a meal or drink clean water. They valued what they had and were grateful for it. It was a humbling experience that taught me that true happiness comes from within and that gratitude is the key to a fulfilling life.

In Haiti, I found a deeper meaning to life, one that revolved around giving, appreciation, and gratitude. It was a reminder that happiness is not just a destination but also a journey, and that journey begins in my mind.

Several years later, I was training at a large chain fitness center. On my way to use the restroom, I passed by a room with some sort of group class taking place. On the other side of the glass was a dark room filled with about a dozen women. The one who caught my attention was closest to the glass. She was sweating while lying peacefully on a floor mat placed under her back, with her face up and eyes closed. After using the restroom, I walked past the room again on the way out. The class had just finished and the ladies were walking out. There she was, coming right toward me. We glanced at each other and smiled.

"Hey, what kind of class was that? You're all glistening."

"Oh, it's Ashtanga vinyasa yoga. It's physically demanding, but it's so rewarding. I feel amazing after each class."

"That sounds intense. I've never tried yoga before, but maybe I should give it a shot."

"Definitely! It's every Sunday. You should come to one of the classes sometime."

"Sounds good. Thank you. By the way, my name's Will."

"I'm Maya. Nice to meet you, Will."

We exchanged phone numbers and continued chatting for a few more minutes before saying good-bye. As I walked away, I couldn't help but feel excited about the possibility of trying out this new class and getting to know Maya better. Who knew what could come of it?

That same day, I went out to purchase yoga gear, excited about seeing her at the next class or maybe sooner. She didn't return my attempts to contact her and we didn't see each other again. I was glad we'd met. That interaction was what it took to finally get me to start an incredible new journey. It completely changed my life. I haven't missed many yoga classes since that day.

My attraction to the opposite sex planted the seed for my yogi journey. Time would reveal it was deeper than just finding another hurdle to put in front of the Grim Reaper.

Although I wasn't sitting like I had during my earlier desk job phase, my rear was still planted on chairs too much. Whether it was time spent behind the wheel or at a computer, writing, I felt my back was paying the price. It was an uncomfortable price I was no longer willing to pay. Occasional back spasms would command my full attention and ruin any plans I might have set for the day. I'd seen too many people around me suffer from chronic back pain to follow the same path. As a personal trainer, I knew how important the spine was in maintaining good posture and promoting a youthful appearance. Spinal disks may degenerate with age, but certain habits accelerate the process.

I started to attend weekly yoga classes at different locations of the same fitness center. It was like learning another language. Not only was my body transforming but the instructors used many words I wasn't familiar with. They all spoke about *asanas*. After class, I found out they were referring to specific yoga poses and how they were designed to improve spinal health, flexibility, and strength. Other times they talked about *prana,* or flow of energy. In yoga, the spine is seen as the main channel for energy to flow throughout the entire body. I was responding well to the Downward-Facing Dog (*Adho Mukha Svanasana*), Cat-Cow (*Marjaryasana-Bitilasana*), and Child Pose (*Bhujangasana*). I was also learning to keep my poise while staying still in extremely uncomfortable positions. This was made possible through intentional breathing (*pranayama*). Circulation blockages I may have had went away.

Within weeks, I saw my range of motion improve and felt tension and tightness dissipate from my back, shoulders, legs, and other areas. My posture became so much better. It was as if I had gained an additional inch in height.

As I was writing this, I peeked at the clock and noticed I'd become totally unaware of time. One hour went by quickly. Being productive feels good. Happiness is contributing in ways that make me feel whole. Writing has provided that feeling ever since I can remember. I imagine movement without limitation or borders. That's the freedom in which my pen moves or my fingers tap on the keyboard. It's a medium where I can gather my experiences and express them in meaningful ways. Whenever my mind is engaged in a thought-provoking activity like writing, I feel internal happiness. Nothing else matters when the attempt to formulate a sentence to express a particular thought is in progress. My hands are in constant motion, tapping letters on the keyboard. At times, it's still pen to paper. Writing can be stressful, too. Externally, the focused facial expression may appear to be frustration. It's a different type of stress when you receive gratification during the process. Every completed idea is an accomplishment. Each paragraph and chapter accumulate toward the goal of completion. My breathing is relaxed. Writing is a sport, but I can't recall ever breaking a sweat—not even when a dozen-page paper was due the next day in college. The pressure motivated this one-time master procrastinator to produce solid work. I don't like sitting in one place for too long, so getting up to move around is must for me. To anyone who doesn't know me, the stern, focused expression on my face may suggest that I am holding a grudge with the pen and pad or laptop. There's nothing further from the truth. I'm the definition of happiness when engaging in these activities.

> **GEM:** It took me a while to figure out that most happy posts on social media are examples of people faking happiness. Exaggerations of success and alterations to improve one's beauty are the norm. I felt like I wasn't living up to my potential. While there's always room to improve, I was

comparing my life to the lives of people I would probably never meet. Once I dedicated time away from social media and focused on myself and loved ones, I began making tremendous progress toward personal goals—one of which was finishing this book.

Over time, I discovered a common link between the activities I enjoyed and the positive vibes. Happiness didn't come from just doing these activities; it came from progress. The more I excelled, the more I wanted to continue. That feeling of accomplishment was temporarily satisfying. It lasted just long enough for me to want to do it better the next time. Measurable improvements increased my confidence. The chemicals released in our bodies when we're happy have been known to ease physical pain and help increase our life spans by several years.

I've had a job or two that I was content with, but I never had a job or obtained a degree that provided me with happiness. Joy is something that comes from within. I used to compare myself to other people. Now I can laugh at myself and shake my head. It's funny how shallow my thinking was. I never saw beyond what I was focused on. In many ways that was a good trait. But comparison to others only led to depressive thoughts. That reasoning was a result of distractions. It came from forgetting and/or not knowing what I was here to contribute. My purpose on this planet is different. I lost sight of what it was. I became disorientated with who I was. At some point I realized that there will never be another me. Wisdom taught me that patience on this unique journey is necessary. It wasn't until I became confident standing in my shoes and fully committing to a manifestation of a vision that my reality would change.

In college, I was a binge drinker. Every weekend, a few of my fellow students and I would go to the local bars. If they didn't ID us, we'd push our internal organs to the brink of alcoholic exhaustion. I never liked the taste of beer. In fact, it was downright nasty, especially the longer the beer was exposed to room temperature. I drank because everyone else who did appeared to be happy. Who doesn't want to be happy with everyone else? Alcohol also gave me beer muscles, a temporary feeling of invincibility that assisted me in building up the courage to talk to random girls. As fun as it may have been to ride the highs, the crashes were brutal. There were many nights where my body accelerated the evacuation of alcohol through every orifice. I learned the hard way that it didn't belong in my body.

Years later, I worked in the tasting rooms of various wineries on the North Fork of Long Island. By that time, I had given up all alcoholic drinks. Yes, I was a proud quitter. That was impossible for many of the people I met out there to believe, especially my coworkers. The access to free swigs of craft beers and bottles of wine was their main motivation. I couldn't have cared less. My purpose was to get myself out of my comfort zone by being forced to talk to people I'd never met. Something told me that whatever I ended up doing in the future would rely on that skill. Being an introvert by nature, I felt that I wasn't exploiting certain talents. Opportunities to network were lost because it was easier for me not to engage. The fear of rejection was an illusion in my mind that I had to tackle. The other reason I decided to get behind the bar was the money. Whatever I wanted to do in the future would also require capital. As time went on, I became more comfortable doing both. Was I happy? In some ways, yes. I loved the fast-paced environment. Moving around and looking people in the eye helped to improve my confidence in social situations. Remembering drink orders helped strengthen my memory. Having conversations about a great variety of subjects was incredible. I met some great people who came from all over the world. They were professionals, celebrities, blue-collar workers, Wall Street types, and everything in between. Some of us had even made genuine connections that proved to be long-lasting. Live musicians often played popular cover songs, which attracted larger crowds. And on those days, I got to listen to great music and count bills hand over fist all night. I'd started to learn the basics of investing, so I knew what to do after those windfall nights. Eventually, I completed my first book, *Quake,* and it opened up an incredible opportunity for me to connect with readers who were interested in my story. I became known as the author behind the bar, and those interactions meant the world to me. It felt strange being asked to sign copies of a book I'd written, reminding me of the times I stood in long lines at the local comic-book store when I was a teenager, asking the author or illustrator to sign my comic book. Now I was on the other end. But I wanted to pursue a bigger passion. After several hours behind the bar, I turned down offers to hit other wineries and bars with my coworkers. Drinking alcohol after busting my ass behind the bar seemed pointless. Instead, I became certified as a personal trainer and holistic sports health consultant and practitioner. I felt a new sense of purpose and a responsibility to at least be who I said I was. What was the point in promoting myself as a health coach if I wasn't healthy myself? Reading health and wellness books and articles took up most of my free time. If I wasn't doing that, I was either training myself or other clients to get in better shape.

I noticed that many of my coworkers would call in sick or show up with baggage from their life outside the bar. They were unhappy, despite all the access to free booze one could imagine. They were attempting to drink away pain, just like I used to do in college. I was years older than most of the staff and had applied learned principles in order to kick the bad habit. The buzz from the alcohol became so addictive that many of them would drink while on their shifts. On the weekends, we'd start at 11:00 A.M. and they'd begin with their first drink to break their fast. The more I researched health, the more I felt like a fish out of water. At first, it was cool to hand people drinks and watch their faces light up with smiles. But minutes later, they'd be puking it back out in the bathrooms or, even worse, on themselves. Compared to earlier, the look on their faces when the buzz wore off was like night and day. It got to the point where I could meet people I'd never seen before and tell what part of the state, country, or world they were from. They didn't even have to open their mouths. I was also able to tell if they had a drinking problem. The distinct lines on their faces spoke volumes before they said a word. The regular customers would visit multiple times a week. With their member discounts, they'd purchase glasses, bottles, and cases of wine each and every week. Some would age decades in the several years we came in contact. Consistent alcohol consumption is an express ride to premature aging. Wrinkles, dry skin, puffiness, red cheeks, and purple capillaries under the skin are all obvious signs of a heavy drinker. It's all fun and games when the drinks are flowing and the band is playing, but when the music stops, reality sets in. At times, it became sad to watch.

I witnessed couples who appeared to be in love in the spring file for divorce in the winter. Women who laughed with one another like they were the best of friends would say the nastiest things behind their backs. The smiles that appeared after a taste of alcohol could easily be mistaken for joy. No. Patience revealed the reality that the smiles were attempts to mask the unhappiness inside.

I've learned a great deal from all the environments I've been fortunate to be in. Happiness for me is being aware of my gifts and using them to positively impact others. It's finding a challenge in fun activities that I can do all day, every day with or without financial gain. Happiness is being comfortable shining my light without having to outshine others. For me, being happy does not always have to be expressed with a smile. It can be a feeling of contentment. It can be an energy felt by others in an unspoken language. Happiness is peace of mind. I have experienced many moments of happiness. I look forward to enjoying many more. Having said that, I do not feel like it's possible for me to be happy all the time. The current state of the country I'm living in and the condition of the world around me are always cause for concern. Maybe I'll address those issues in another creative medium. Being present and fully engaged with who and what brings fulfillment is the road I'm on. I'm enjoying the ride.

14

SOLAR SYMPHONY: DANCING WITH THE ENERGY OF LIFE

With every rising of the sun, think of your life as just begun.
— *Anonymous*

From the moment I could comprehend the world around me, the sun became a source of endless fascination. Whether it was flipping through the pages of *Odyssey* science magazines as a young boy or breaking down the sun's various layers for my fifth-grade science project, I was driven by an insatiable desire to understand its secrets. The image of what appeared to be an orange fireball above the clouds always captured my full attention. Was it really orange, or were those scattered particles that appeared orange? Either way, the sun was the ultimate symbol of power and life to me.

News reports I watched on the television would warn about the dangers of excessive exposure to its powerful rays. Especially, when the UV index, a measure of the level of ultraviolet radiation, was high. Meteorologists always advised against spending more than fifteen to twenty minutes in direct sunlight. They said it would age our skin prematurely and increase the chances of melanoma, a form of skin cancer. The dark spots on the skin of people diagnosed with this disease would scare me. Dermatologists would use these images for their ad campaigns. I'd see them in magazines, television commercials, even on bus and train posters. My first year of college in Miami, Florida, started during a sizzling summer. Ninety-degree temperatures there felt different. The hot conditions took some time to adapt to. The high humidity outside made it feel like I was wearing an extra twenty pounds on my back. Never had I experienced heat like that before. A few people walking on the streets held umbrellas to shield themselves from the hot sun. Most of them had skin darker than mine. I guess they didn't want to get any darker. Before long, I found myself doing the same as I walked to and from classes. Yes, I really did hold an umbrella over my head when it wasn't raining.

I remembered an experience at an outdoor swimming pool one August afternoon. It had been months since I had been out in the sun. Some friends and I decided to cool off by having a small pool party. The UV index was at its highest level, and the humidity was almost unbearable. There wasn't a visible cloud in the sky. We gathered around the pool, music playing in the background, and drinks in hand. I had my shirt off, and I swam for hours. The water felt refreshing as we splashed around, laughing and enjoying one another's company. I felt invincible. Certainly the water would provide protection from the scorching sun shining directly over my head. I was wrong.

A few hours later, I noticed that my skin was starting to feel tight and hot. I ignored it, thinking it was just the heat, but I soon realized that I had gotten a sunburn for the first time in my life. My friends noticed my discomfort and urged me to go inside and cool off. I applied aloe vera, but the damage was already done. I spent the rest of the day indoors, nursing my sunburn. I didn't understand why my skin became tender to the slightest touch later that day. The sun reflecting off the water only accelerated its intensity. I learned a painful yet valuable lesson that day. Much later, I understood why my skin burned. Sunburn was my body's response to excess toxins being brought to the surface by the sunlight. During this time dead food options were in heavy rotation on my daily menu. Toxic blood was being brought to the surface to be cleaned and eliminated at an accelerated rate. My skin turning from caramel to red was a gentle warning signal. Nature was sending me a message that my skin wasn't ready for intense sun. The overly processed foods I indulged in sure didn't help. I didn't wear any suntan lotion then and I haven't since. At first it was because no one with dark skin around me did. Later it was because I didn't want any chemicals to block my skin's ability to burn. It didn't make sense to apply a barrier between my skin and the sun, reducing the absorption of beneficial rays. I made some lifestyle adjustments and began to feel the rays stimulate immunity in my body. It felt better than when I would take a pain reliever to block the sensation of pain for temporary relief. Not addressing the cause of the pain eventually led to nagging injuries and continuous consequences. Trial and error taught me to address major causes by adding more colorful fruits and vegetables to my plate at each meal. Gradually, I was able to increase my time in the sun and tan safely without getting burned again. The colors in the produce I eat are a result of antioxidant pigments called anthocyanins. In the plant kingdom, these powerful pigments protect against pests and other stressors, such as intense sun. With bounteous amounts of bright-colored produce on my plate came the protections against many of my previous health issues.

As I delved deeper into my journey toward better health, I realized that I needed to take a cue from nature itself. The plants around me swayed and thrived under the warm embrace of the sun, and it dawned on me that I, too, needed this radiant energy to nourish my body. The sun wasn't just a celestial object in the sky; it was also a vital source of sustenance for my very being. I learned that sunlight catalyzed the production of calcitriol, also known as vitamin D, in my skin. This hormone played a critical role in maintaining my overall well-being. Without it, my bloodstream would be choked with impurities, and I'd be a sorry sight indeed. But calcitriol was much more than a mere filter for my blood. It helped me fend off infections, fortified my bones, balanced my hormones, and even kept my mental health on an even keel.

It was a revelation that left me stunned. Hormones were the lifeblood of my existence, yet I couldn't find them in any food. They were within me, and they needed sunlight to thrive. The realization hit me like a bolt from the blue: I needed the sun to maintain my youth.

I'd always heard that fifteen to twenty minutes of sunlight was enough to fulfill my daily vitamin D requirements. It was a piece of advice that had been drilled into my mind by the mainstream media for decades. But I soon realized that this recommendation was tailored for people with fair skin. My skin had more melanin, and that meant that I needed much more time in the sun to kick-start the synthesis of calcitriol. It was a startling revelation that completely changed my outlook on life. I wasn't just a passive observer of my surroundings; I was an integral part of the world around me. My body and mind were connected to the environment in ways I'd never imagined. As I basked in the warm glow of the sun, I knew that I was on the right path toward better health and a brighter future.

Throughout the years, I couldn't help but notice the peculiar behaviors of my overweight and obese coworkers. They shied away from the sun as if it were their worst enemy, and they avoided live, edible plants like the plague. It was almost as if they were disconnected from the world around them, existing in a bubble of lethargy and poor health.

As I began to undergo my own transformation, I gained the confidence to observe these patterns more closely. It was a consistent cycle of staying indoors during sunny days, keeping comfort foods and snacks within arm's reach, and avoiding any form of physical activity. It was no surprise that these individuals were more prone to sickness, recurring injuries, and frequent mood swings. Intrigued by this connection between their dis-ease, compromised immune systems, and lack of sunlight, I dug deeper into the science behind it all. It was then that I discovered the significance of sunlight energy, stored in the nucleus of cells as biophotons, for optimal health.

I started to soak up the sun as much as I could, exposing my skin directly to its healing rays. By consuming more plants that absorb energy from the sun during the process of photosynthesis, I was getting more energy indirectly. Biophotons help connect all living things on this planet. With each passing day, I felt an increased sense of connectivity with the world around me. The more I consumed living foods, the more I felt like a part of the natural world. I even started having more vivid dreams, some in color, some in black and white. And if I had to interrupt my dreams to answer nature's call, I could often remember the details upon returning to sleep, as if I'd hit a mental pause button.

It was almost as if I had tapped into some hidden universal energy source. I felt a heightened sense of awareness, more in tune with nature than ever before. And in some strange, inexplicable way, the world seemed to respond to my newfound energy. People I hadn't spoken to in ages would suddenly call me out of the blue, and I would find myself meeting strangers I had previously only thought about. It was as if I had unlocked the secrets of the universe through my journey toward better health. And as I continued to explore the fascinating world of biophotons and living foods, I knew that I was just scratching the surface of what was possible.

Complex societal puzzles were becoming easier for me to simplify. Increased fat cells contribute to vitamin D deficiency. With the rising rates of obesity, I noticed around me, it began to make sense. The nutritional infrastructure influenced by the fraudulent food pyramids I was taught in school has not benefited the ever-increasing number of sick people. My diet had a huge impact on how much sun I could safely consume. Dead animals, packaged foods high in salt and chemicals, artificial sugars, alcohol, drugs, etc., did not protect me from getting burned. Identifying these harmful sources was key for me. No matter what a person's skin tone, the sun will bring the toxins within up to the surface of the skin. High amounts of toxins from unhealthy sources always eventually lead to some expression of dis-ease. Consistently consuming dark, leafy greens and colorful fruits make it much easier to reap the many benefits the sun has to offer.

GEMS: I increased my ability to extract energy from the sun and safely stay out longer in it by eating more fresh, whole plants. As the lines of communication with the sun improved organically, it became easier to know instinctively how much sun exposure was necessary. Whenever I see young, healthy people, they tend to have a surplus of energy. Sharing this energy in a positive way maintains balance and improves our environment. The natural, sustained energy I have is a direct result of my relationship with the sun. Dead animals and overly processed foods do not offer the biophotons I need to exist harmoniously with nature. The disconnect we are currently experiencing with the rest of the universe is largely due to the low levels of biophotons among humans.

15

YOUTH REDISCOVERED: BALANCING RESPONSIBILITIES AND DREAMS

When your friends begin to flatter you on how young you look, it's a sure sign you're getting old.
— *Mark Twain*

In my youth, I was a carefree child, unburdened by the weight of responsibilities and concerns that come with adulthood. I remember watching a story on the news that left a profound impact on me. It was about twin boys who were born with a rare genetic disorder called progeria. These boys, who were around the same age as I was, looked like they were fifty years older than they actually were. Their skin was wrinkled, they had lost all their hair, and their youthful appearance had vanished. Progeria is a progressive disorder that causes children to age rapidly, starting from their first two years of life. Progeria, Greek for "prematurely aging," didn't allow most children with it to live beyond thirteen years, twenty at the most. That made it clear to me why the disorder was rarely passed down in families.

The disorder robbed them of the joys of childhood, leaving little time for them to build lasting memories, establish friendships, or dream about their future as adults. I couldn't fathom what it would be like to age two or three times faster than my parents, and the thought of it was terrifying. It was clear why the boys were being filmed at a Disney theme park. Time was fleeting for them, and they were eager to experience the ultimate childhood adventure.

As I grew older, my perception of time changed. The abundance of youth that once consumed me became something to manage. I reminisced about the days when my friends and I played stickball in the streets of Long Island. We were carefree and independent, stopping everything to retrieve the ball, which was the key to continuing the game. Winning and impressing our peers meant everything, and we talked about great plays for weeks, even years.

But as responsibilities and bills began to pile up, the stakes became higher. Money started to play a bigger role, not because it could buy time, but because it could give me more control over how I spent my time. As an adult, I was still a grown-up kid, and my moves became more calculated to meet my responsibilities. Whenever I was able to stop everything and retrieve the ball, financial compensation was usually involved. Although the stakes are higher as an adult, the rewards for pursuing better health and well-being are priceless.

> **GEMS:** Consistently eating foods that require the least amount of energy for the body to digest has proved to be a great way to help me prevent premature aging. Foods such as water-rich fruits and nonstarchy vegetables have allowed my body's organs to work efficiently while being able to free more energy for healing and other daily activities.

The high water and fiber content in these foods supports clearing out toxins before they can stress my systems. My energy feels more sustained and consistent throughout the day when my diet centers on produce. In addition to the physical effects, this way of eating has shifted my mental state as well. My mood is consistent and my thinking clearer. With each bite of fresh produce, I'm literally investing in my future self - contributing to my healthspan as well as lifespan.

16

BLACK DON'T CRACK: DECODING THE MYTHS AND REALITIES OF AGELESS BEAUTY

Race is the child of racism, not the father.
— *Ta-Nehisi Coates*

The moment I heard the phrase "Black don't crack," my curiosity was piqued. Could the color of my skin hold the key to defying the ravages of time? Was there a secret antiaging formula woven into my DNA, accessible only to those with melanin-rich complexions? Perhaps darker skin possessed a sort of superhuman ability, capable of slowing down the inevitable march of aging. Could it be possible? I couldn't help but wonder.

This topic wasn't brought to my attention in school. Well into my adulthood, my curiosity led me to research. According to the khanacademy.org website: "Between 70,000 and 100,000 years ago, *Homo sapiens* began migrating from the African continent and populating parts of

Europe and Asia." Modern man first emerged from Africa, and we are all descendants. The scientists conclude: "When humans migrated from Africa to colder climates, they made clothing out of animal skins and constructed fires to keep themselves warm; often, they burned fires continuously through the winter. Sophisticated weapons, such as spears and bows and arrows, allowed them to kill large mammals efficiently."

As humans migrated farther from the Earth's equator, the need for melanin to protect against the sun's harmful UV rays decreased. This gradual shift away from tropical regions ultimately resulted in lighter skin tones. While I've always had a natural sweet tooth for fresh fruits, it's important to note that humans were primarily fruit eaters before venturing into colder, less hospitable regions. As vegetation grew scarce in higher latitudes, humans were forced to adapt and hunt animals for sustenance, mimicking the behavior of carnivorous animals. This practice would become increasingly common over time. As humanity continued to evolve, numerous other differences began to emerge.

Dr. Llaila Afrika writes in his book *African Holistic Health*, "Blacks have specific biochemical, nutritional and dietary needs. These nutritional needs arise because blacks are melanin dominant and have specific bodily differences as compared to less melanated races. For example, over 70% of black people (worldwide) cannot digest cattle milk. In addition, the intestinal florae (bacteria, virus, fungus, and yeast) that naturally live in black people's intestines are unique to blacks."

Instinctively, I always knew that all humans come from the same source. We share many similarities and have phenotypic differences due to the ways we have adapted to climate, geography, and overall environment. Black people in North America have had an extremely difficult time adapting to their environment, which was transformed during the tenth century. Instead, they have been conditioned to conform to standards of systematic European colonization. The biases within the race-based society we live in do not favor the differences between Blacks and others. As a result, Black people are often misdiagnosed and misguided by the medical system. Black people have not benefited under the Western medical system's demand for quantifiable data as evidence of effectiveness. A system that understands and appreciates the unique needs and differences of every individual, and works to address them, rather than trying to force everyone into the same mold, is missing.

I was skeptical of modern medicine and the chemicals that came along with it. So when doctors told me I was vitamin D–deficient, I wasn't too keen on the idea of taking a vitamin D shot or pill. Living in New York, I was aware of the drastic decline in sunlight's strength and duration after the summer months, which can lead to a deficiency in the vitamin. But I refused to subject myself to experimental chemicals and injections, which were being thrown around too freely for my liking.

Whenever I asked about the ingredients of these vitamin D supplements, I was met with blank stares or visible frustration. It was as if the mere suggestion of questioning what was being put into my body was a crime. But I wasn't willing to take that risk unless it was a matter of life or death. After all, these doctors didn't even know what, exactly, was in the substances they were injecting or prescribing. It was a game of Russian roulette, and I wasn't willing to play.

I also began to read historic articles and realized that the medical system as a whole didn't benefit Black people. I knew that vitamin D, which is really a hormone, is produced whenever our skin is exposed to direct sun rays. One of the most obvious phenotypical differences between Caucasian people and Black people is the darkness of the latter's skin. I read in *The New England Journal of Medicine* that although vitamin D–binding proteins are lower in Blacks, this doesn't result in increased bone fractures. The article concluded: "To improve the determination of vitamin D status in diverse populations, the measurement of vitamin D–binding protein will most likely need to be incorporated into the assessment."

Most Black people I've spoken with over the years have told me they were taking over-the-counter vitamin D supplements or getting vitamin D injections from their doctors. Vitamin D deficiency is especially common among dark-skinned people living in northern latitudes. This leaves them vulnerable to weakened immunity, seasonal affective disorder, other forms of depression, and various cancers. Dark-skinned people can thrive in high sunlight environments if they embrace the sun and consume mostly plants. By conforming to European standards of working indoors from 9:00 A.M. to 5:00 P.M., exposure to the sun during the peak hours of 10:00 A.M. to 4:00 P.M. is lost, especially during the winter months.

Whenever I made more effort to increase my exposure to the sun, I always felt more energized— as long as I didn't try to get too much too quickly. I began to realize that my body had the ability to absorb sunlight in the summer and reserve it throughout the winter. The results were undeniable. Each time I returned to the same doctors for tests, my results showed significant improvement. The signs of deficiency were gone, and I felt stronger and more vibrant. It was clear that the key to my health and vitality was in understanding my unique biological needs and embracing them fully.

I was born into a global system that separates people into different races. The concept of race did not exist before it was created by Europeans. François Bernier's 1684 publication, "A New Division of the Earth by the Different Species or 'Races' of Man that Inhabit It," is often credited as being the first articulation of race theory. In the 1700s, Carl Linnaeus and Johann Friedrich Blumenbach's human-categorization ideologies started to gain more widespread acceptance among Europeans. During the eighteenth and nineteenth centuries, the social construct of race became institutionalized. The theory of people with dark skin being inferior to Caucasians was used to justify the enslavement of Africans for the purpose of denying basic human rights and obtaining free labor. Audrey Smedley's newsletter entitled "Origin of the Idea of Race" states, "From its inception separateness and inequality was what 'race' was all about. The attributes of inferior race status came to be applied to free blacks as well as slaves. In this way, 'race' was configured as an autonomous new mechanism of social differentiation that transcended the slave condition and persisted as a form of social identity long after slavery ended." More recently, the American Society of Human Genetics explained, "The science of genetics demonstrates that humans cannot be divided into biologically distinct subcategories."

For a few seasons, I tended bar at a jazz lounge. I couldn't help but notice the reverence for youthfulness among the predominantly Black crowd. One of the regular live performers onstage would tease the birthday and marriage celebrants, claiming they couldn't possibly be older than twenty-five. The crowd would erupt in laughter and cheers, playing along with the game. But beyond the lighthearted banter, I saw a deeper fascination with the supposed age-defying properties of melanated skin. They sounded sincere when they told me how healthy they were. Their fancy jewelry and designer wardrobes looked impressive, but I couldn't find much evidence to support their claims of being healthy. According to the Centers for Disease Control and Prevention's website, "Black women are disproportionately burdened with obesity. An estimated 80% are overweight or obese." My own observations would confirm this information to be accurate. These numbers were from 2019 and may be even higher by the time this book is published. People with chronic diseases would come to the bar to celebrate after their doctors gave them a "clean bill of health" based on blood test results. I would ask myself how one can be healthy with symptoms of chronic disease. The simple answer is, it's impossible. Misinformation is often easier to find than the truth.

The bar for good health has ingredients to make greens salads, not Long Island ice teas. At times, I felt uncomfortable bringing people instant gratification, knowing the later results would not be as positive. They had been so far removed from the core principles of their origin that they no longer understood what true health was. Millions of years ago, African people thrived on mostly fresh plants. Animals were eaten occasionally and made up a small portion of the diet. This was new information for me, too. Years ago, fruits and vegetables were local, sustainable, and organic. Before World War II, organic simply meant from the earth. Today, I see organic foods with their own section in supermarkets. A 2012 article available at sciencedaily.com examined teeth from the skeletal remains of hominins found in a South African cave dated to be almost two million years old. Researchers used dental picks and laser devices to determine the foods eaten. The article states, "This gives us a very clear picture of their diet, and it was surprising. It shows that they ate more fruits and leaves than any other hominin fossil ever examined, more like what a chimp might eat." That article led to my discovery that bonobos are the closest living relatives to humans. There's a 98.7 percent match in DNA. They also consume mostly fruit, leaves, honey, small vertebrates, and other primates whenever plants are not available.

When I looked at the Trans-Atlantic Slave Trade Database, it estimated that 10.7 out of 12.5 million Africans survived the Middle Passage and disembarked in North America, the Caribbean, and South America. These were mainly West Africans, who ate a predominantly vegetarian diet, centered around rice, okra, yams, peas, peppers, and millet. Meat may have been used sparingly as a seasoning. Africans were not only forcibly separated from their land, families, and culture, they were forced to eat against their will on the slave ships. Chisels and hammers were used to break through the teeth of those who refused. Funnels were used to pour food down their throats, through the holes created by the chisels. Some African staples were brought on the ships and even planted in the plantation fields wherever they landed. After the slave masters ate, they gave the slaves scraps of pig's feet, ribs, intestines, neck, liver, head, and other undesired cuts that would be rationed each week. Black people turned to creativity in times of despair and transformed whatever they were given into more palatable dishes. These poor nutrient-value meals became a tradition known as soul food. Today, the modern SAD (standard American diet) of factory farm–raised animal products, dairy, and processed foodlike substances has taken tremendous tolls on health. The people most negatively affected are Blacks in the Americas and other continents around the world.

Malcolm X's words still resonate today: "When white folks catch a cold, black folks get pneumonia." For centuries, Black people have been grappling with the devastating consequences of economic and health disparities. Chronic stress has taken a toll on many, leading to hypertension, premature aging, and even death. The damage wrought by 2020 and beyond is yet to be fully understood, but one thing is clear: The disparities will only worsen in the coming years. Tainted water supplies in Flint, Michigan; Milwaukee, Wisconsin; Jackson, Mississippi; Baltimore, Maryland; and Chicago, Illinois, are just a few examples of environmental racism. Ironically, Flint, Michigan, is only a five-hour drive away from Lake Superior, the largest body of fresh water in the country. Black neighborhoods also remain in the grips of food apartheid, with limited access to fresh produce and supermarkets often miles away. Fast-food restaurants, liquor stores, and bodegas, on the other hand, are ubiquitous. This systemic injustice has deprived Black people of the crucial phytonutrients, antioxidants, vitamins, polyphenols, micronutrients, minerals, fibers, and other anticancer plant compounds that are essential for good health. The inadequate consumption of these vital nutrients has been linked to increased levels of depression, mood disorders, anxiety disorders, and even suicidal thoughts. The struggles and challenges that Black people face in their daily lives are a reflection of a larger problem, one that must be tackled head-on if we are to create a more just and equitable society.

During my conversations with Black people at the bar where I worked, it was evident that they often assumed themselves to be in good health if they had not received a formal medical diagnosis of an illness or condition. Even if they had visited a doctor recently, it was common for them to forgo medical attention unless they were experiencing a visible injury or severe pain. This attitude may stem from the historical and ongoing struggles in Black communities, which have endured atrocities and continue to face hate crimes and systemic injustices. For Black people, every day is a battle in a treacherous maze of a society that relentlessly targets and discriminates against them, making each step feel like a survival game against deadly obstacles.

Surviving in a system designed to separate individuals from their freedom and opportunities is already a daunting task, and it becomes even more challenging when one's true identity must be concealed to secure a coveted corporate position. The scarcity of such opportunities further intensifies the struggle for those who strive to thrive in a world that is not always welcoming to their authentic selves. The toll of this systemic racism on mental and physical health can be significant, even as some Black individuals celebrate each milestone decade of life.

It is remarkable that Black individuals do not appear decades older when one considers the trials and tribulations they have endured. While stress can take years off one's life, the false perception of good health among Black people is a concerning issue, one that warrants attention.

Over the years, I have observed mainstream media and medical professionals promote Botox and collagen injections as a "cure" for wrinkles. During my research into the significance of collagens, I discovered their crucial role in providing structure and elasticity not just to the skin but also to bones and other areas of the body. What surprised me was their vital function as a natural shield against the sun's harmful UV rays, particularly in darker skin.

It is a common misconception that applying collagen and elastin topically can provide the same benefits. However, my research has led me to the realization that the molecular structure of these proteins is too large to penetrate the skin's surface, making their topical application useless. To make matters worse, some skin-care products contain penetration enhancers, which facilitate the infiltration of harmful toxins into the skin.

This revelation was alarming and made me more cautious about the products I used. During my research, I read online articles featuring skin specialists and aestheticians. They explained that Black skin's high oil content and sebaceous activity contribute to its natural hydration system, which keeps it looking hydrated, smoother, and plumper, resulting in a slower aging process.

Reflecting on my findings, I realized the importance of understanding the science behind skin-care products and their effects on our skin. Prioritizing natural hydration methods and avoiding harmful toxins that can cause irreversible damage to our skin is crucial for maintaining healthy and youthful-looking skin.

Throughout the years, I have received numerous compliments about my youthful appearance. Some people attribute it to "good genes," while others suggest that having children could potentially change my appearance. While these factors may have some influence on how one ages, it is important to note that they are not the sole determinants. In my observation, I have seen parents who develop full heads of gray hair by the time they reach forty, and former star athletes who gain a significant amount of body fat within months after retiring from professional life. While genetics do play a role, it is essential to acknowledge that one's lifestyle habits can have a much greater impact on physical appearance.

Harmful habits such as a lack of physical activity, poor dietary choices, and smoking can accelerate the aging process and contribute to a decline in health. Additionally, exposure to environmental factors such as pollution and UV radiation can damage the skin and lead to premature aging. Therefore, it is crucial to adopt healthy lifestyle habits in order to maintain a youthful appearance and overall well-being. This includes engaging in regular exercise, eating a balanced diet, protecting oneself from harmful environmental factors, and avoiding harmful substances. While genetics do play a role, each of us has the power to control our lifestyle choices and ultimately impact our aging process.

An article written in the *Los Angeles Times* said, "Fewer black people are able to sleep for the recommended six to nine nightly hours than any other ethnic group in the United States. . . . Poor sleep has cascading effects on racial health disparities, including increased risk of diabetes and cardiovascular disease." The article goes on to say, "The racial sleep gap is largely a matter of unequal access to safe, reliable and comfortable sleep environments . . ." On March 13, 2020, Breonna Taylor, a twenty-six-year-old aspiring nurse, was shot to death by police in Louisville, Kentucky. She was in bed, sleeping in her own apartment. The police, looking for drugs, barged through her front door without knocking and fired their weapons. The Jefferson County Coroner's Office released Breonna's autopsy report. She was struck six times. The fatal bullet struck near her heart, tearing through her main pulmonary artery connecting her heart and lungs. Breonna Taylor was not the suspect on the warrant. No drugs were found in her apartment. At the time of this writing, the four race soldiers who committed this brutal murder have been charged but not arrested. The psychological disturbances from events like these can affect a population of people indefinitely. Imagine hearing a noise in the middle of the night after absorbing this horrific story. This is one of numerous examples of why even sleeping while Black has never been easy in America.

Homo Sapiens is not a perfect species. I'm like everyone else because I was born with certain traits that run in my family. My body has certain areas with imperfect characteristics, much like a weak link in a chain. These weak links or genetic predispositions can leave me more vulnerable to certain symptoms of dis-ease. Life experience has taught me how to strengthen these imperfections. Some people have organs that can withstand more abuse than those of the average person. Others need organ transplants earlier in life. Like myself, most Black people I've encountered don't trust the current healthcare system. Males are especially wary of the system. That biannual checkup they recommend will most likely end up happening one to three years later, if at all. That's only if the doctor's office calls and/or sends constant reminders. Going extended periods without addressing a problem can result in diseases that go undetected and worsen over time. But the long history of mistreatment of and heinous acts against Black people provides enough motivation to begin seeking alternative routes.

There are numerous examples throughout history that detail reasons for Black people's mistrust. One of the events that impacted me the most was what occurred from 1932 to 1972. I came across one of the most unethical medical experiments in American history: the Tuskegee Study of Untreated Syphilis in the Negro Male. Conducted by the United States Public Health Service, this diabolical study involved six hundred African American sharecroppers from Macon County, Alabama. They were all twenty-five years old or older, and extremely poor. Out of the 600 participants, 399 tested positive for syphilis, a sexually transmitted disease.

When I dug further, I discovered that in exchange for their participation, the participants were promised free health care, meals, and burial insurance by the federal government. They were told that the study would last only six months, but it went on for a whopping forty years! The participants did not give their informed consent to be used as research subjects, and were promised a cure that never came. Instead, their disease was left untreated, and they were told that they were being treated for "bad blood," a term used to describe anemia, syphilis, and fatigue.

A chemical called penicillin was standard treatment for syphilis during that time, but the researchers were more interested in watching the progression of the disease in the men. It is incredibly disheartening to learn that the main causes of death for Black people in the southern United States were cardiovascular diseases back then. Not much has changed.

I also found a disturbing story that occurred in 1972 regarding the Tuskegee Study. Peter Buxtun, a whistle-blower, brought the unethical study to light by speaking to the press, which ultimately caused the forty-year experiment to end. Shockingly, seventy-four of the participants were still alive at that time. Out of the 399 male participants with syphilis, 28 of them suffered from the disease until they died, while 100 others died from related complications. Additionally, forty wives of the participants were infected, and nineteen of their children were born with congenital syphilis. This study was considered to represent a national health crisis at the time. The aftermath of the Tuskegee Study was devastating.

It took sixty-five years, until 1997, for the White House to issue an apology for the Tuskegee Study. Survivors like Herman Shaw, who was thirty years old at the start of the experiment and ninety-five in 1997, were present when the apology was made. Shaw stated that "the damage done by the Tuskegee Study is much deeper than the wounds many of us may have suffered. It speaks to our faith in government and the ability of medical science to serve as a force for good. We were treated unfairly—to some extent like guinea pigs. We were not pigs.... We were all hardworking men and not boys ... and citizens of the United States. The wounds that were inflicted upon us cannot be undone. I'm saddened today to think of those who did not survive and whose families will forever live with the knowledge that their deaths and suffering was preventable."

The families of the survivors were able to reach a settlement with the U.S. government for ten million dollars. They were misled by the United States Public Health Service, whose name was later changed to the United States Department of Health and Human Services (HHS). Essentially, these two organizations are one and the same. Today, the Centers for Disease Control and Prevention (CDC) is a federal agency under the HHS and operates as the nation's leading public health agency. The Tuskegee Study is a tragic reminder of the unethical practices that can occur within medical research. The impact it has had on individuals and their families has lasted generations.

I witnessed the global lockdowns of 2020 further highlight the inequalities facing Black people. As the racial wealth gap increased, I saw Black communities suffer yet again from misinformation, unhealthy lifestyles, and inadequate access to organized health and wellness solutions due to systemic disparities.

The disparities in life expectancy and disease mortality rates for Black individuals living in the United States are concerning. According to the National Vital Statistics Reports, in 2017, the white population had a life expectancy of 78.6 years, while the Black population had a life expectancy of only 75.3 years. These figures have only worsened in the wake of the global lockdowns of 2020, with Black men experiencing a life expectancy of under sixty-eight years and Black women one of seventy-five years. In contrast, white women had a life expectancy of 80 years and Hispanic women 81.3 years.

Furthermore, I discovered that in Haiti, where both of my parents were born, the Institut Haïtien de Statistiques et d'Informatique (IHSI) reported an average life expectancy of just sixty-four years. These findings underscore the need for further research and action to address health disparities and promote health equity.

It is important to note that the inequalities in health care are a result of the systemic racism that Black people have endured for centuries. The government's and media outlets' unprecedented push of experimental chemicals to address public health crises was astounding, leading to widespread skepticism and distrust among Black people. The mistrust of the health-care system will continue as younger generations are educated about the systemic injustices their ancestors faced. According to the CDC, African Americans between the ages of thirty-five and sixty-four are 50 percent more likely to have high blood pressure than whites. The same website also reveals that African Americans are more likely to die at an early age from all causes, including cancer, high blood pressure, type 2 diabetes, and stroke. These statistics are alarming and highlight the urgent need to address the underlying factors contributing to these health disparities. If humans share approximately 99.6% - 99.9% of their genetic code with one another, it must be the growing wealth and resource disparities that continue to fuel these negative trends. The fight for health and economic equity must continue until everyone, regardless of race or ethnicity, has equal access to quality health care and the resources needed to lead healthy lives.

Black people are undoubtedly one of the most resilient populations in the world. The devastating impact of the Middle Passage and slavery disrupted their cultural practices and tore apart families. However, through the years, Black people have exhibited remarkable strength and perseverance. To reverse much of the damage inflicted upon them, proper health education and a return to a more natural way of life could prove to be effective. By addressing the root causes of premature deaths, such as violence within the community, economic inequality, and police brutality, we can begin to eradicate systemic racism and create a more just society.

It is worth noting that most chronic diseases that disproportionately affect Black individuals, such as cancer, type 2 diabetes, HIV/AIDS, stroke, and high blood pressure, can be prevented or even reversed through nutritional and lifestyle changes. When the body lacks the necessary nutrients to handle stress, it can become worn down, leading to accelerated signs of aging.

The younger generations now have access to a wealth of information on portable and virtual computer devices, including long-term, peer-reviewed studies with hard end points. My hope is that books like this one will spark greater awareness and curiosity, inspiring individuals to take control of their health and well-being. By embracing a holistic approach to health, one that addresses physical, emotional, and environmental factors, we can promote longevity and vitality among Black individuals. It is through this collective effort that we can continue to celebrate the resilience of Black people and honor their enduring legacy.

So where did I meet my largest case-study groups? At the bar. What were they doing? Drinking alcohol with artificial sweeteners, eating heavily salted, greasy, genetically modified dead animals and processed foods, smoking cigarettes and cigars, and vaping toxic chemicals. All of this while waxing poetic about how "Black don't crack." The dim lights of nightlife, thick, full-coverage makeup, hookah and cigar smoke, and mirrors are deceptive. They can easily hide cracks from free-radical damage to the untrained eye. But upon further inspection, patrons were suffering from one or more health conditions. Dozens told me they took chemicals for high-blood pressure, type 2 diabetes, cholesterol, and other complications from obesity. Others endured long bouts of recovery from surgical procedures (hip and knee replacements, organ transplants, heart operations, and cataract removal). Many Black people are extremely sick but have become great at hiding their symptoms in order to survive. I did notice an increasing interest in menu items that were labeled "veggie." Was this because the term had become trendy? Were they aware of their impact on the Earth's rapidly changing climate? Had they seen the videos of the unnecessary cruelty done to animals? I wasn't sure. I was just happy to see their conscious efforts to move toward what was marketed as healthier. Eating fresh plants, engaging in vigorous exercise, getting lots of rest and adequate sunlight, drinking clean water, and spending time in the fresh air seemed extreme whenever I was asked about my regimen. It's that lifestyle that has allowed me to recover my health. To them, I was a freak of nature. I was just imitating people I'd read about or interacted with, those who functioned like I wanted to function. Anyone I've consulted who followed these steps has responded favorably, too. I didn't get the impression the bar patrons understood the harm they were inflicting on themselves each week. It became crystal clear that the effects of dietary choices on health was a confusing topic for many people. It was obvious to me that their lifestyles in and outside of the bar had starring roles in their declining health.

I've always assumed that the phrase "Black don't crack" refers to Black people who don't look like they've suffered much in the way of hardships. In actuality, Black people have continuously endured the worst health conditions and fought against the toughest odds in the most hostile environments. The illogical reality of Black inferiority and the constant terrors of systemic racism influence all areas of human endeavor. These weapons have been pointed in the same direction with laser-beam focus for hundreds of years. They have taught Black people how to normalize stress. I fully support speaking truth to power. But the expression "Black don't crack" has provided a false sense of security. Repeat it like "abracadabra" and, poof, good health will suddenly appear. No. That hasn't been my experience at all. I know how consistent I had to be to earn better health. I had to make it a priority. Health is what makes all other things possible. The mistrust of the modern medical system is warranted. The health-care disparities are criminal. There are too many examples of institutions not serving the best interest of the oppressed. The responsibility lies with the people to research holistic health and emphasize self-care. When Black people exercise on a consistent basis, drink clean water, breathe fresh air outdoors regularly, secure the right amount of sleep, absorb adequate rays from the sun, and eat mostly minimally processed plants from the earth, something magical happens. They don't crack.

17
YEAR OF THE RETURN: A HOMECOMING CELEBRATION

If I have ever seen magic, it has been in Africa.
— *John Hemingway*

Two thousand nineteen marked four hundred years since the first enslaved Africans were brought to the English colony of Hampton, Virginia. The Ghanaian government encouraged the African diaspora to visit, settle, and invest in the country during what was called the "Year of the Return." As soon as my feet touched the soil of Ghana for the first time, every single cell in my body celebrated with joy. It was similar to the feeling I got whenever I arrived in Haiti, but this felt different. There was a distinctive magnetic pull. My brother, nephew, and I all felt it. I was curious to see what Western miseducation systems had been trying to shield from me. The history books in schools I attended were notorious for reinforcing false narratives about Africa. I was taught to expect primitive people, thick jungles, and lack of resources. The capital city of Accra was the total opposite. It felt like home.

As we got into the Uber, the driver greeted us warmly and asked where we wanted to go. "We're heading to the hotel," I replied, looking out the window as we made our way through the bustling streets. It was impossible not to notice the throngs of Ghanaians walking around in the hot sun, going about their daily business. "Man, people sure love to exercise here," my nephew remarked.

I nodded in agreement, but then my expression turned serious. "You know, I read about how American fast-food chains are popping up in other African countries. It's a real shame."

The driver couldn't help but agree. "Yeah, it's one thing to read about it, but it's another thing to see it firsthand." As we drove by a "Murder King" and a "Kentucky Fried Cancer" restaurant, I felt a pang of sadness. "Look at all these places. It's like they're everywhere."

But amid all the chain restaurants, there were also plenty of independent entrepreneurs who had set up their own fast-food-style eateries. "Check out all these signs for jollof rice and fried chicken," I said, pointing them out. "It's like they're on every corner."

"Well, let me tell you, these fast-food joints are popping up everywhere in Ghana and across the continent. It's the latest trend, especially among the young and middle-aged Ghanaians. They see it as a symbol of status, you know? Like, they want to identify with the images they see of Western culture. If you're eating at a fast-food restaurant, it means you're in tune with the latest trends, and that's where the cool, hip crowd hangs out. But of course, you gotta have some extra cash to spare, because fast food is a bit pricier than traditional cuisine."

"Wow, I never thought of fast food that way," my nephew said.

"So where do the locals go for traditional cuisine?" I asked.

"Oh, there are plenty of options for traditional cuisine. You can try some of the local food joints or even some of the street vendors. They're all over the place. And trust me, the food is amazing!"

"That sounds great! We'll have to try some of that, too," my brother said.

We checked into the hotel, dropped our bags in the rooms, found a restaurant across the street to eat at, and crashed for the night.

The next morning, as the soft light of the sun started to peek over the horizon, I rolled out of bed, battling the grip of jet lag. Despite the exhaustion that tugged at my eyelids, I had to reclaim my body's natural circadian rhythm. Stepping out of my room, I made my way to the hotel's front lobby, where there was a small, gated courtyard. The moon hung low in the sky, casting a pale ethereal glow over the tranquil space. I began to move, my body gradually awakening as I performed calisthenics beneath the light of the moon.

Suddenly, a voice broke the stillness of the morning.

"Good morning. Excellent day for exercise," the voice of Carnaval, the hotel manager, echoed through the courtyard.

"Yes, it is," I replied.

As Carnaval opened the gate to go outside, I couldn't help but wonder why I was the only other person up at this time. It was a serene and peaceful atmosphere that you rarely experience in a busy city. An hour later, as the first rays of sunlight began to pierce the sky, Carnaval returned, his energy undiminished, and joined my family and me at the breakfast table.

"How safe is this area?" I asked, wanting to ensure that we were in a secure location.

"Every morning I run before five. Would you all like to join me tomorrow?" Carnaval responded enthusiastically.

"That's way too early for me," my brother said, yawning.

"Yeah, I don't think I can make it, but you guys have fun," my nephew said, smiling.

"I'll need a day to recover from our flight," I interjected. "But after that, let's do it!" I exclaimed, feeling motivated by Carnaval's energy.

"Okay," Carnaval replied, his tone unwavering. "Whenever you're ready, I'll meet you in the lobby at four-thirty."

The next day, as the city slumbered and before the street vendors set up, Carnaval and I were already on the move. The air was crisp and cool, and the silence was only broken by the sound of our footsteps pounding the pavement. With a quick stretch, we set off on our daily pilgrimage, a four-to-five-mile run that would invigorate our bodies and our spirits. Carnaval was an inspiring professional soccer player who also understood the importance of staying in shape.

As we jogged along the streets, he was like a guide, leading the way and warning me of any obstacles that might trip me up. He was intimately familiar with every manhole-size drain along our route, and he deftly steered me clear of them. I couldn't help but marvel at their depth, which seemed to rival those I had seen in Port-au-Prince, Haiti.

Suddenly, a deep, guttural sound interrupted our rhythm. I looked around, puzzled, trying to pinpoint the source of the noise. Carnaval chuckled and shook his head. "Those are frogs," he said, as if it were the most obvious thing in the world.

"Frogs?" I repeated incredulously. "That loud? They sound like big animals."

He nodded. "Yes, many people eat them, especially in the north."

As we continued our run, the burping sounds of the frogs became a familiar background melody, a symphony of nature that accompanied us on our journey. With each step, I felt myself becoming more attuned to the world around me, more alive and more connected. It was a small, simple moment, but it stayed with me long after our run was over.

This was the first time in my adult life when I didn't feel the need to look over my shoulder for crooked cops. I'd be naïve to think that corruption didn't exist. But racist white cops didn't work here. Self-hating Black cops eager to uphold a white power structure? Maybe. This was the honeymoon phase, but I didn't see any evidence of that, either. The tension in my muscles began to relax more each day. The natives knew I wasn't Ghanaian, but I didn't feel targeted. I felt respected and embraced as a member of the human family. It wasn't a crime to explore my surroundings and enjoy nature. I'm sure the chats I'd previously had with those who'd traveled here before had something to do with preparing me for these moments. But to actually experience this was pure bliss. The positive energy was contagious in the best way possible. I've seen so many people die prematurely under pressure. High blood pressure is a silent sniper that takes the lives of hundreds of thousands annually. My circadian rhythms calibrated nicely in this environment. Dreams appeared more frequently. My quality of sleep improved with each night. I couldn't help but weigh the pros and cons of continuing to live in the States.

I was beyond excited to take in the scenery before the hustle and bustle. We had been in Ghana for a few days. I noticed something I had never witnessed before. I had to ask.

"Where are all the elderly people? Even in the daytime I don't see too many."

"They stay inside their homes."

"What's wrong with them?"

"Many of them don't feel comfortable outside when it gets too busy."

"That's too bad."

"They don't want to fall or get hurt."

Weeks earlier, I'd read a book on Africa my nephew gave me. It detailed the continent's emerging economy. It also highlighted a unique demographic. Statistica.com reported that Africa has the youngest population in the world. On the flip side, it also has the world's lowest life expectancy. In West Africa, males, on average, live fifty-six years and females fifty-eight years. In 2019, the life expectancy in Ghana was sixty-four years.

In the distance, I heard the faint sound of chanting growing louder. Curious, I turned my gaze toward the source of the commotion. A group of about a dozen kids emerged from the horizon, jogging in single file with unwavering discipline. Clad in vibrant soccer jerseys, shorts, and cleats adorned with the colors of Ghana—red, yellow, green, and black—these young athletes moved with a sense of purpose that was both awe-inspiring and humbling.

The leader of the pack couldn't have been older than ten, yet he commanded the group with confidence, leading kids who were even younger. They greeted us with a unified call and response in Twi, one of the main dialects of Ghana. *"Maakye!"* they exclaimed in unison, wishing us a good morning. *"Yaa anua,"* Carnaval replied.

As I watched these children, I couldn't help but wonder if they were truly just children or if they were adults in young bodies. Their level of dedication and passion for exercise was remarkable. During my own upbringing, early mornings were often spent rushing to the hospital due to asthma attacks. But here, these children were up before the sun, driven by a desire to represent Ghana in soccer someday.

I realized that these kids were not just moving physically; they were also exercising freedoms that many adults took for granted. They were seizing the privilege to dream and chase after their visions with unbridled enthusiasm. It was a stark contrast to what I was used to seeing in my regular environment—broken children trapped in adult bodies. These young athletes were embracing the opportunities life had to offer outside of their comfort zones, just like I was.

As we ran, I found myself sweating and my heart pounding in my chest, just like the kids beside me. We shared a common curiosity to experience life to the fullest, to explore the unknown, and to push ourselves beyond our limits. It didn't matter our age; the rewards of exercise were equally gratifying, reminding me that the pursuit of health and vitality transcends generational boundaries.

After our run, I retreated to my room to shower and prepare for breakfast. I turned on the television, and a health program caught my attention. A panel of so-called experts was discussing the dire state of health in Ghana at a global health convention. Malaria, stroke, HIV/AIDS, diarrheal diseases, diabetes, and ischemic heart disease were the leading causes of death in the country, these experts said. Malnutrition, poor diet, alcohol, high blood pressure, lack of exercise, and unsafe sex were cited as some of the main contributing factors.

I was taken aback by this revelation. Everywhere I had been in Ghana, I had been struck by the country's natural beauty and abundant resources. Yet the people on the panel, representing renowned international organizations, were visibly overweight and seemed disconnected from the realities of the population they were discussing. It was a sobering reminder that unhealthy lifestyles and decision making by individuals and organizations can have detrimental effects on the health of communities they are meant to serve.

It was becoming clear to me that Ghana, like many other places in the world, face health challenges that require holistic and comprehensive approaches. It isn't enough just to acknowledge the problems; resources focused in the right direction are needed to make changes at both individual and societal levels. I realized that there was much more to learn and uncover on this beautiful continent. The adventure had just begun, and I was eager to know more about the mysteries of Ghana, its people, and its quest for health and vitality. The Aburi Botanical Gardens were a paradise of lush greenery and vibrant colors. As we drove up the steep, winding road toward the mountain, I felt like I was on a thrilling roller coaster. Our first stop was at a local farm stand, where we picked up some juicy coconuts, watermelons, pineapples, and mangoes. The fresh fruits were a burst of flavor and sweetness that I had never tasted before.

As we entered the gardens, I was mesmerized by the vast array of flora and fauna surrounding us. Dozens of bird species I had never seen before were chirping sweet melodies above us. The rich red clay soil was bursting with life, and I couldn't help but wonder what stories these ancient trees had to tell.

We met Maxwell, a knowledgeable guide, who told us about the various trees and plants in the gardens. He introduced us to the true cinnamon tree, and we had the opportunity to scrape some fresh cinnamon off its inner bark. I was shocked that I'd never known that this was where the real cinnamon came from. It was coveted for its antioxidant properties and benefits for slowing down the aging of the brain. This sweet, woody flavor was nothing like the cinnamon I had grown up consuming in processed breakfast cereals, candies, and chewing gums.

Maxwell also pointed out the abundance of fresh cocoa on the trees, informing us that Ghana was the second-largest producer of cocoa in the world. I had eaten refined chocolate my whole life—in chocolate milk, cookies, cereals, cakes, ice creams, shakes, candy bars, and more. But this was my first time eating the actual fresh fruit, and I was blown away by its soft, tart white flesh. This was the purest form of chocolate, known for its beneficial properties for improving brain function and gut health.

My journey to Africa was a transformative experience in many ways. It shifted my perspective on culture, food, and life in general. The trip to the

Aburi Botanical Gardens was particularly eye-opening, as I tasted the original sources of flavors that I had known only in processed forms. However, my excitement for the future was tempered by concerns about the rise of Western fast food in African countries. Looking at the devastating effects of this trend in the United States, I worry about the impact it will have on African populations already struggling with malnutrition, disease, and other issues stemming from resource disparities. What will African countries look like as their populations are expected to undergo rapid growth? African countries already rank among the lowest when it comes to life expectancy. Unhealthy eating trends will only make a bad situation worse. I'm all too familiar with the addictive nature of certain foods and their disastrous impact. Nevertheless, I look forward to returning to Ghana and other countries to learn, share, and experience the energy of the motherland.

GEMS: For years, I struggled to understand why so many African countries were among those with the lowest life expectancy globally. The biggest industries in the world rely on Africa's abundant natural resources. With incredibly fertile farmland, how could its people suffer from malnutrition and die so prematurely? Why are there no "blue zones" in Africa? By all accounts, Africans should enjoy the highest global life expectancy.

The truth became clear once I walked the land and spoke with its people. The misconceptions I had been taught - that Africa was "undeveloped" before European colonization - were false. In fact, African civilizations, societies, cultures, technologies, sciences, agriculture, trade, and governance were thriving long before Europeans arrived.

Today's high rates of respiratory infections, HIV/AIDS, diarrhea, malaria, perinatal conditions, measles, and other diseases largely stem from the unequal distribution of wealth and resources on the world's most resource-rich continent.

YOUNG @ ANY AGE

18

SOLE SEARCHING: DISCOVERING ABILITY WHERE I LEAST EXPECTED

The battles that count aren't the ones for gold medals. The struggles within yourself—the invisible, inevitable battles inside all of us—that's where it's at.
— Jesse Owens

Any activity that required me to run was always tough. Daily bouts with bronchitis as a kid kept my airways blocked, lungs constricted, nose stuffy with mucus, cough consistent, and a foggy feeling in my head. These symptoms were worse during the colder fall and winter seasons. On occasion I used an inhaler to ease the tightness in my chest. Running was no fun when I couldn't breathe without wheezing. I had to run at some point in order to play soccer, basketball, football, and kickball in grade school. The nature of these sports provided momentary breaks during time-outs, halftime, and other stoppage of play—especially basketball. A random pause was just enough to divert thought away from the fatigue that kept knocking on my conscious mind. I always admired track and field from afar. I feared having to be judged solely for my ability to run a certain time or clear a specific distance. I knew my cardiovascular weaknesses would be exposed every time. What was the point in even trying?

I started to take running more seriously much later. After watching the NYC marathon on television around 2009, I started to pay attention. Crossing the finish line with a smile after running five- or six-minute miles for 26.2 miles? That's what the runners from Kenya and Ethiopia did. Wow! I became intrigued with the preparation necessary to complete one of the most impressive human feats. I didn't have it in mind to compete with top runners. It was the thrill of completing a challenging goal that caught my attention. Running offers numerous challenges. You won't feel the same during every run. One day, you might have to deal with a sore toe. The next day, the knee you hyperextended the week before may throb slightly every quarter mile. If you slept wrong, your neck may affect your posture, etc. For me, the feeling of fulfillment after a grueling run has been rewarding every time. So much so that it may take some effort to revisit how hard it was during the run. I guess that's the long-lasting effect of adrenaline rush. I slowly began to incorporate outdoor running into my fitness routine. My body welcomed the test. Once it became a habit, I started thinking about more ways I could stay young, fit, and make a living at the same time.

Personal training seemed like a sensible transition. A flexible schedule and active lifestyle became priorities for me. In order to become eligible to train in gyms, I had to pass an exam to get certified. I took a six-week course at Farmingdale State College in 2011. A dozen of us sat in a classroom with desks and chairs on one side and gym equipment on the other. The instructor was in his early thirties. I was a few years older. As knowledgeable as he was about human anatomy and physiology, and training, his philosophy on nutrition was the opposite of what I was learning through my online holistic nutrition class. Over the next few weeks, I became acquainted with some of the other students. During breaks in the class, we shared some of our goals as well as our backgrounds. As the weeks went by, the class would chuckle and watch me writhe in discomfort as the instructor gave his thoughts on nutrition. He told us how important it was to eat lean meats and dairy, especially right after a training session. He agreed with the textbooks that these were the best sources of protein and calcium.

He also told us that running was one of the worst exercises. It was supposedly bad for our joints, especially our knees. He showed us a scar from knee surgery he'd had years earlier. He had injured himself while running. After that, he vowed never to run again. Once more, I heard playful giggles from some students in the class. It must have been entertaining to watch me shaking my head in disagreement. A few students and I had talked during an earlier break about how I had been running outdoors. I ran a couple of miles five times a week. My joints felt better than they had in high school, where I played multiple sports.

Is physical wear and tear a factor as we age? Sure it is, but the reason this instructor said that running is bad for the knees is because he was miseducated. The pain and discomfort that I've felt at times in my joints are real. Beginners and weekend warriors are more likely to experience soreness and pain from stressing dormant parts of the body. The true cause of pain and the solution is not as well known. Evaluation would need to be done on a case-by-case basis. Experience has taught me that sports injuries can be caused by multiple factors. Poor running mechanics, improper footwear, tight muscles, and insufficient rest are common among new runners. This does not make running a bad exercise.

> **GEMS:** Stretching for a few minutes at the same time each day has helped me to not accelerate the aging process. By simply setting an alarm on my mobile device, I can create a habit of breathing deeply while performing a handful of stretches. I may not like to stretch, but improving flexibility makes everything else easier.

Author and researcher Robin Hur wrote this in an article entitled "Osteoporosis: The Key to Aging": "All animal products are high in chlorine and sulfur, low in manganese and magnesium, and with notable exceptions, they are high in fat and low in vitamin C. Surprisingly, every one of these characteristics tends to impair bone development and/or retention."

My observations led me to conclude that most of the damage to my joints as well as my lungs was being done internally as a result of poor nutrition. Animal products and overprocessed foods were the main culprits all along. They were the main cause of the debilitating joint issues so many people around me suffered from. Robin Hur also wrote, "The ties between animal products and the entire 'aging' process (i.e., the transfer of calcium from the bones to the soft tissues), and osteoporosis in particular, make the cornerstone of the 'four basic food groups' look like a tombstone. Normal diets contain enough protein to produce rapid bone loss even among young adults. They also contain enough phosphorus to cause debilitating bone deterioration; and they have a calcium-to-phosphorus ratio that would be expected to both thwart bone development and speed deterioration."

Some people move with noticeably bad form, have poor posture, and lack flexibility. These deficiencies can make bodily damage worse over time. I taught myself how to move through repetition. My knee issues as a kid weren't so much a result of wear and tear from pounding the pavement. They came mainly from the same foods I was now being trained to recommend to my future clients. I kept thinking to myself, How did earlier man survive out in the wild? Why did man evolve to standing upright on two bare feet? What did humans do thousands of years ago, before they created weapons and encountered danger? It seemed to me that running was one of the most natural movements for a human being. As challenging as it was, I decided to keep quiet in my seat. We were all in that classroom to prepare for the exam. The classes were at least four hours long. Each time we met, we went through several chapters of course work. The reason I was taking this class was to get the certification I needed to be a personal trainer. In order to pass the PT exam, I had to regurgitate the words the instructor repeated from the books. It hurt me to have to answer questions with information I knew was wrong. As much as I may have wanted to, it wasn't the time to debate.

In 2019, I was doing personal training at a gym in Florida. I met Terrance, a new client, who was coming off of a long layoff from training. Years of constant sitting in an office and hour-long commutes to and from work had taken their toll. We trained for hours each week. He understood the importance of staying consistent with training on our off days. This is where most personal training clients fail. I'm sure most trainers will agree. After six weeks, he was one of the fittest members at the gym. Other trainers and gym goers noticed. He mentioned he had completed multiple marathons. We talked about the training it took and the thrill of completion. Unbeknownst to him, he was now my running coach. I had confidence that his résumé would help me accomplish a longtime goal. Although Florida is a predominantly flat peninsula, we ran on hills at a park that was once a busy landfill. Its 65-foot mound is one of the highest elevations in southeast Florida. The hills were rocky and steep, and the experiences were awesome. The challenge was that we were meeting only once per week. That meant I would have to be consistent all of the other days—just like he was when I was training him. Any trainer with an ounce of passion wants the people he's trying to help to give it their all: full commitment and the willingness to work hard. It was time for me to walk it like I talk it. I promised to put in the work and see how my body responded.

I went out and bought an activity-tracker watch to monitor my heart rate and distance. I began running a minimum of twenty miles per week. Running provided a tremendous opportunity for me to release stress and combat the effects of stagnation. I could think clearly about whatever was going on in my life without distractions. Shortly after, Terrance asked me to run with him in a local 5K event. I agreed to join him and participate in my first 5k.

I made sure to get at least eight hours of sleep the night before. On race day, I was well rested. Between 150 and 200 runners showed up. We walked to the start line to await the gun. A ninety-year-old man would do the honors. He stood with good posture, cracked jokes with onlookers, and appeared to be in great shape. My heart pounded with nervous energy. "On your mark, get set..." he yelled. Then he pulled the trigger. Terrance was gone in a flash. Many of the other runners whizzed right by me within seconds. A few of them had heads full of gray hair. I didn't want my ego to write a check I couldn't cash. My training had been consistent but nowhere near the pace of these other runners. I found my feet moving faster than normal. I had to remind myself that lots of energy would be needed for the finish line. That goal was still three miles away. Halfway into the race, I began to pass a few of the runners who had sped by me earlier. As I suspected, they'd started too fast and now were running out of steam. I knew I was doing well, because I had never felt this fatigued for this long during my training sessions. With one mile remaining, I tried to keep my pace to the finish. As I approached the finish line, the crowd of spectators started to yell words of encouragement. That motivation gave me a boost of belief and I finished at a faster pace than when I'd started the race. I ran a personal best of 24:03. I'd trained for several months and had never run faster than thirty minutes! Terrance and I both finished second in our age groups.

After the race, we went to a board where the final results were posted. It listed the categories, runners' names, hometowns, finishing times, and ages. As fast as I thought I'd run, there were three males sixty-five and over who'd run faster. I'd caught a glimpse of them at the starting line, before they took off and left me in the dust. I checked the times to confirm. One male was seventy-seven, and he'd crossed the finish almost a full minute before I had. I kept thinking back to what that personal training instructor had said about running being a horrible exercise. I'd known he was wrong then, but this event further confirmed that. Not only did I feel the difference but I was in the presence of others who were living it.

I had watched a video on YouTube about a former Navy SEAL. He talked about how he had once weighed over three hundred pounds and became disgusted with how he looked and felt. Inspiration from the Rocky films inspired him to try to join the military. After years of hard work, he ended up completing marathons and ultramarathons. The guy's story of overcoming hardship after hardship was amazing. He was in his early forties but appeared at least a decade younger. In another video, he was receiving top honors at a Navy SEALs' ceremony. He broke down in tears when trying to describe to those in attendance the sacrifices his mother had made for him. My eyes got watery just watching this. I noticed he was the only man in the entire room who looked like he could still run a mile without collapsing. I later found out that years after his military retirement, he still runs several miles and trains daily. He was quoted as saying, "When your mind is telling you that you cannot possibly go any further, you're only actually 40% done." What I heard in those videos resonated with me. My normal morning routine up until that point was to get up and run three miles a day, which I did five days a week. The morning after watching the David Goggins video, I got up and ran five miles. I've made that my new minimum ever since.

The following spring, Terrance and I decided to skip the 10K (6.2 miles) and attempt my first 15K (9.3 miles). Sounded great. But wait . . . I had never completed more than six miles without stopping before. Once the event date was set, we began to work on fifty- and one-hundred-yard sprints to develop more speed. I stayed consistent with five-mile runs and pushed to six miles whenever time allowed. A few weeks before the race, I felt pain in one of my knees every day. Doubts started to creep in my mind. Maybe my instructor had been right. Was wear and tear finally catching up with me? I started taking multiple days off, something I wasn't used to doing. After three days, I'd go out and test the knee again and the twinge would welcome me back with sharp lightning strikes of pain. Terrance and I decided just to focus on finishing the race and not going for time.

YOUNG @ ANY AGE

It was March 7, 2020. Race day was finally here. I felt all right, but a poor decision to bartend the night before had kept me up later than originally planned. A handful of hours later, we drove to Marathon, Florida. Over four hundred runners were attending this event. The butterflies were stationed in my stomach. This was far bigger than the 5K. It was also twenty degrees cooler and breezy. Good temperature for a run but only when moving with the wind. We were surprised to find out that after completing a 10K, we'd have to stop and wait for all the runners to finish. Then we'd line up at the start again to run a 5K. It was disappointing that the 15K was separated in this way, but we were already there and decided to make the most of the event. When the start gun sounded, runners shot out and took off. I kept my cool and stayed at around the pace I'd been running while preparing for this day. I knew it was better not to go out too fast. Maybe it was the adrenaline rush, but I didn't feel any pain in my knees. Once again, I looked up and saw the backs of runners with gray hair and athletic postures. A few miles in, I felt the urge to urinate. Perfect timing. Now I'd have to try and block that out of my mind for another four miles. Easy, right? Terrance passed some of the runners who had taken off at speeds faster than they were able to maintain. I knew that he was running way slower than he was accustomed to doing. I saw what he was doing and liked the strategy. Good plan—once we pass, they stay behind us, I told myself. To keep pace, I did the same. It was comforting to hear the sounds of music from their headphones slowly fading in the distance. I used each runner we passed as a small victory to fuel my mind to stay the course. The pants of labored breathing and heavy feet skipping the ground diminished with each step. The smell of musty cologne began to lessen with each stride forward. I tried to take my mind off of the pain in my legs by trying to guess familiar scents. I may have had a bottle of that fragrance, I thought. Smells like a light green tea. I remember that it came in a clear bottle. Was it Joop? No, it was CK One. I wore that just about every other day. Definitely before heading out to the nightclubs, but not before working out. Cologne doesn't mix well with sweat. There. For about sixty seconds I was able to trick my mind into thinking about something other than the stress I was putting my body through.

The next runner Terrance decided to pass was a middle-aged woman. I could tell that this wasn't her first running competition. Her pace was steady and we were already moving faster than I was used to after four miles. I wanted to let Terrance know I didn't think this was a good idea. But he had already begun to pass her, and I was too tired to speak without yelling. I reluctantly followed his lead. It took a lot of energy for me to keep up with that move. Unlike my experience with the other runners we had passed earlier, I didn't hear her footsteps fading away. Without looking back, I was able to feel her determination to keep up with us. I knew, because I wouldn't like getting passed at this stage of a race, either. Great. Now I'd have to keep this pace for at least another mile and a half. I was struggling to keep the easy, free form with which we'd begun the race. I looked up at the overcast sky and started searching for a reason to quit. My lungs were beginning to burn, my legs felt heavier, and the wind kept gusting. What did I just get myself into? Was it obvious that I was beginning to lose steam? I wanted to slow down, but doing so would relinquish the lead we'd worked so hard to achieve. I was laboring to keep pace. Terrance was still cruising effortlessly in low gear.

I had been training consistently but nowhere near as hard as I was pushing myself now. This was uncomfortable approaching unbearable. My heart was thumping, my legs were blazing, and my abdomen was cramping from holding back the urge to urinate for so long. The closer we got to the finish line, the more people lined up along the side to cheer on their friends and family. Each time I heard the footsteps behind me get louder, I somehow found a way to run a little faster. The ultimate letdown would be to work so hard to get the lead, then give it back with the end so close. I kept telling myself to relax. This was only a dream. This was only a light jog. Nothing near what my legs were telling me. After bending around the final curve, I could see the finish line in the distance. We were about three hundred yards away. The footsteps behind us were getting faster and louder. "We're almost there. Let's go!" Terrance said before darting ahead. The one-hundred-yard sprints on the high school football field would have to kick in now. I gave it all I had and took noticeably longer strides. I couldn't hear any footsteps other than my own. The cheers blended in with the wind until the moment we crossed the finish line. Terrance finished the 10K portion of the event at 51:09. I came in at 51:10, seventeen minutes faster than I'd ever run.

It took ten minutes to catch my breath and finally use the restroom. Running that fast for another 3.1 miles (the 5K portion of the event) would not have been possible for me that day. A voice behind me said, "You guys brought out the best in me back there. That was my fastest run this year." When I turned around. I saw it was the middle-aged woman. "We brought out the best in each other. That was a great run," I replied, giving her a high five. She confirmed that what I'd felt earlier was indeed a truly competitive spirit. Human energy is a contagious phenomenon. Terrance and I jogged super slowly around the beach area and stretched in attempts to keep warm. I was physically spent and losing the motivation to continue with the 5K portion. We'd end up waiting another fifteen minutes for the 5K to start. We agreed to run with no expectations. After twenty-five minutes, the 5K was about to start. I usually recover quickly after a run. But after pushing so hard, my legs were cooked.

There were more runners at the line this time. The 5K was half the distance, and more of the younger runners participated. I looked around and noticed new, fresh faces and dry short-sleeved shirts. The sun was rising and the temperature was warming up. When the gun sounded this time, we jogged lightly as runners passed us by. Of course, some of them were decades older. They hadn't received the memo that they were old and running on pavement is "bad" for the knees. My joints felt great, as well. The farther we ran, the more runners we passed. I told Terrance to slow down several times. I was beyond tired. I looked up at the clouds in the baby blue sky, trying as much as possible to keep from hunching forward. As we approached the halfway mark, Terrance looked over and said, "Only a mile and a half left. This'll be over soon!"

"Not soon enough," I mumbled, barely able to form a sentence.

Once more, there were footsteps coming from behind. We were holding them off, but they stayed close enough for me to hear. As the finish line came into view, Terrance said, "We're almost there. Let's move!"

I spotted two runners ahead who looked like they were fading fast. The orange cones on the side of the road near the finish were in plain view. I passed one of the runners with about one hundred yards to go. I was redlining my body. I had to decide whether or not to empty the tank. I started to gain ground on the second runner, who had on ear-covering headphones. Whatever he was listening to had him in another world. He didn't notice how fast I was closing in, with only forty yards to go. I didn't know if it was his support group, but a bunch of people standing along the sidelines got animated and started pointing in my direction. Why can't they just keep quiet? I wondered. He glanced over his left shoulder in complete shock and picked up his speed. During all of my practice runs, I'd made it a point to finish quicker than I'd started. This was literally the moment I had been training for. It was me and him in an all-out sprint. The finish line was an electronic mat underneath an inflatable arch. The black mat was shaped like a speed bump, so I knew I had to step on it correctly to avoid a catastrophic ending. We crossed the line at the same time in a photo finish. There were photographers and supporters behind the line taking photos. They quickly scattered to get out of our way as we came barreling down the narrow, straight path. It was a good thing they did. I had little control moving that fast. I finally came to a stop and continued to walk straight ahead. All I could hear was my heart pounding. It felt like it was beating out of my chest. I had never run that fast for so long. The runner I crossed the line with looked back and we looked at each other, gasping for air and extending our arms for fist bumps. We were too tired to say a word, but the look we gave each other spoke volumes. I knew he'd given everything he had and he knew the same about me. It was a moment of unspoken sportsmanship.

The results came in and were posted on a board. Terrance and I both finished in the top ten. The months of work we'd put in were paying off. I was happy with my performance and welcomed the runner's high that followed. It's a feeling of bliss that can only follow an effort that summons mental and physical stamina. I learn more about myself with each run, whether or not medals are awarded. A potential problem at the beginning of the 15K became another possibility to explore my capabilities. I found the power to strengthen my mind/body connection with focus and determination. The more I ran, the further I was able to push previous concerns away from my conscious mind. It's easy to quit the moment a situation becomes uncomfortable. Running provides me with opportunities to train different parts of my mind and body and overcome difficult tasks. Sharpening this skill set is necessary for me to stay young. I continue to find ways to transfer this prowess into other areas of my life. Who knows? Maybe one day I'll cross the finish with a smile.

> **GEMS:** There can be a fine line between pushing toward a personal best and pushing past the point of no return. Admittedly, I blurred the line. I was satisfied with my preparation leading up to these races. The consistency with my training gave me confidence. It encouraged me to feel good enough to push myself past my normal limits. I knew the risks involved and decided to take them. Checking in with a health-care professional on a regular basis can be a good thing. Such people can help you identify underlying problems you may not be aware of. I was also glad I did my own research on health and fitness. This is important before engaging in vigorous exercise or competitive activities.

19

THE MISEDUCATION OF WILL LOISEAU

There are three things that can't be hidden for long: the sun, the moon, and the truth.
— *Buddha*

Whenever I had a fever or cut my finger in grade school, I was sent to the nurse's office. The nurse would allow me access to Band-Aids, aspirin, and a limited selection of over-the-counter chemicals. If necessary, she'd record my heart rate, take my blood pressure, and provide a bed to lie down on if I had a stomachache. I'd get to rest in her office and eat colorful lollipops, too. There were a few kids who would frequently fake sickness until a parent or guardian came to pick them up. Some of them were trying to avoid other kids, who were waiting to beat them up after school. Others were always looking to miss classes they didn't like. I wasn't as confident in my acting abilities. Besides, my parents worked in New York City and wouldn't leave their jobs to travel more than an hour away, not unless I was dying or for some other urgent reason.

The nurse was the person who helped us with minor discomforts. If a situation required serious medical attention, we were encouraged to see a doctor. I wondered why my tonsils didn't swell and have to be removed, which had happened to some other kids in my class. Why did I think about this? Because they got to miss time at school. Kids were "rewarded" with ice cream and mini wooden spoons whenever they returned. Other than a sore throat, they looked fine. Besides, teachers gave them a pass and didn't call on them to answer questions. I envied the kids who had appendicitis and missed school to have their appendixes removed. I'd listen to classmates say that their doctors told them these body parts weren't a big deal. Why would we possess parts that didn't serve any important function in the body? The kids boasted in class that we could easily live without them. The school nurses and teachers stood in front of our classes and told us the same. Was this true? I understood that we could live without a foot but would not get far without a heart. But they are important in different ways. Were we created with useless body parts that served no good purpose? Something didn't seem right about this.

I can still remember what I was served in the hospital during my extended stay for pneumonia. Each day I got to choose from an assortment of processed meats with condiments, refined grains, sugary drinks, cereal with cow's milk, water, and, yes, ice cream. The nurses and doctors told me that these foods would help me to recover and regain my health. The truth is, my youth, the resilience of my body's immune functions, the increased bed rest, my ability to assimilate the few nutrients in the food, and the stimulation from the chemicals they gave me all helped the symptoms to subside. As a kid, I got the impression that body parts were expendable, like the action figures I role-played with. I used to marvel over the process my classmates went through when they'd break an arm or leg. Sure, it was fun to sign their casts with Magic Markers, but what really intrigued me was the speed of healing. Casts would help keep limbs or joints immobilized and protected. Crutches provided support and balance to make walking easier. Kids would show up to class with a cast and about a month or so later it was scheduled to be cut off. Given the right conditions and enough time, their bodies had the natural ability to heal. That powerful concept was not emphasized in any of my health classes. None of the general practitioners I interacted with ever spoke about this. As I got older, my mind became conditioned to see human organs as interchangeable. I thought that removing body parts from individuals dealing with dis-ease was normal. It was happening all around me, and such practices were celebrated as technological breakthroughs on television. Age is an important factor in any recuperative process. At one time, my body was as elastic as a rubber band. When I was still growing, my body was constantly creating bone and muscle tissues. This enabled my peers and me to heal much faster when we were younger. But I was not exposed to the medical professionals who acknowledged the benefits of natural healing. Without understanding the cause of dis-ease, it was easy for me to keep repeating the process that leads to its symptoms. Barring unforeseen circumstances, aren't body parts designed to last the full life of an individual?

Before diagnostic code readers, auto-repair technicians would use engine stethoscopes and experience to diagnose what was wrong with a vehicle. As technology improved, auto maintenance became easier. Since when did a human heart become disposable, like a car battery? Unlike cars, the design of the modern human body hasn't changed much in hundreds of thousands of years. Human evolution has been going on for millions of years. The healing methods that have been effective for centuries have not been embraced by mainstream medicine. The kids I grew up with who later became parents allowed doctors to remove body parts from their kids without question. My peers and I wanted to be like Steve Austin, the main character of *The Six Million Dollar Man,* one of my favorite television shows from the 1970s. He was an astronaut who suffered a near-fatal flight crash. The doctors performed a classified operation and replaced his damaged parts with bionic body parts. He came out of surgery a cyborg, able to run faster than cheetahs, jump incredible distances, and possessed of superhero strength and abilities.

These days, it no longer takes an extreme circumstance for surgery to be presented to a patient as the first option. Technology has continued to advance, allowing previously complicated procedures to be completed quicker than ever. Does faster always equate to being better? If so, better for whom? Is profit over patience/patients the overriding theme in the modern medical model?

Health was one of my favorite subjects throughout school, even though I felt what I was being told wasn't always accurate. It seemed practical that the healthier you were, the easier it was to enjoy youth. The teachers who taught health rarely appeared healthy themselves, but they were less demanding than other teachers. I didn't feel the nervous energy I felt during math and science classes. The health homework was always simple. If there was any at all, it didn't require much effort for me to complete it on time. As interested as I was in the subject, I didn't get the sense of fulfillment I was looking for. I was not sure how to express what I was seeking, but the feeling of satisfaction was absent. At the collegiate level, the classes were barely any better. There was something in the curriculum that was missing. I didn't have a concrete comprehension of health or disease to describe what this was. I was memorizing outdated textbook information, only to spew it back out during multiple-choice quizzes. I couldn't articulate what I really wanted, so I continued to pass without applying any critical thinking.

Years before graduating from college, I worked with seniors at an assisted living community. I was excited at the opportunity to work in nutritional sciences. A few residents were independent enough to live in their own private rooms. The majority of the residents had roommates and needed wheelchairs, walkers, canes, or nurse assistance to get around.

Leo and June, both in their eighties, were still a couple after fifty years of marriage. Leo always wore solid-colored suits, and June was all about bright-colored dresses and stylish hats. Chronologically, the youngest resident was sixty-five, but biologically it was this pair. They were inseparable. Leo walked with a walker but still stood with tall posture. June used a cane from time to time. They were always sociable and seemed like they were enjoying their later years. Every time they came to the dining room, they would both soak up the attention. Leo would then tell a joke.

"Hey, Will. We're here to try the new restaurant. Have you heard about it?"

"No. What new restaurant, Leo?"

"It's called Karma."

"Karma?"

"There's no menu. You get what you deserve."

He always had a new joke to tell.

"Life's too short not to laugh every day," he'd say often. Leo and June were both good at remembering names. They were regulars at game night, where the residents would play Scrabble, bingo, UNO, Name That Tune, and other games.

As a dietary representative, I was being trained to prepare food and beverage portions, assist some of the residents in choosing from the daily menu, and keep track of food temperatures. Some residents had diet cards with modified menus. Their physicians would stipulate selections that were low in sodium, had no sauces, no dairy, or were sugar-free. I noticed something different with Leo and June. They always ate fruit for lunch, broccoli-onion soup and some type of leafy green vegetable with rice or pasta for dinner. I didn't see the other residents eating this way. One day before dinner, I wanted to know more.

"What keeps you two looking younger than everyone your age? What's your secret?"

"Will, I'll tell you, my secret," Leo said with a serious look on his face. "I've been married for fifty years. I promised June when we got married that whenever we argue, the loser has to walk two miles."

"Wow, that's a long walk."

"Yeah, tell me about it. I've been walking two miles every day for the past fifty years!"

"That explains you, Leo, but how does June look so young?"

He answered with a smile: "That's another secret. Every day for the last fifty years, she's been following me to make sure I really walk the full two miles!"

"He still owes me two miles for yesterday," June said.

"I know, I know, honey."

"So, it's all about keeping the feet moving, huh?" I replied.

"And I make sure we eat our veggies," June said. "Want to know the best part about staying active and eating our fruits and veggies?"

"What's that?"

"Eventually we'll be dead and won't have to do this anymore," June said, laughing.

This couple was fun to talk to. They were always in good spirits despite whatever problems they were going through. They seemed to live in the present moment. That was a quality I didn't encounter often.

Although it was still early in my own journey toward understanding what healthy cuisine was, I knew what healthy wasn't. Memory loss, cancers, heart disease, type 2 diabetes, strokes, etc., were common among the resident population. Every few weeks a resident was taken out on a stretcher and would die in the hospital. The nutrition standards were low and not conducive to health. Even I knew that. I discovered that I lacked the knowledge and administrative power to influence healthier choices. I didn't feel comfortable serving sick people dead foods. The smell of some of the dishes was repulsive; they were loaded with toxic chemicals that I wouldn't put in my body. I was still consuming a less than healthy diet myself, but this experience sparked a new awareness. It made me start questioning what I had to change in my own dietary choices. It didn't take long before I had reached a point where I felt it was time to move on.

When I became a certified personal trainer, I learned a lot working with adults. My favorites were the ones with drive and motivation to tackle their fitness goals. Some of their stories were shocking to me. One woman looked like a bodybuilder in her gym membership identification card photo taken several years earlier. She was now in her early forties and looked like a totally different person when I met her. She was 310 pounds when we checked her weight on the scale. Her body-fat percentage was almost 40 percent! She told me that it had been years since her last training session. The desire to push herself athletically was no longer there. She needed me to hold her accountable each week and design a plan for her to follow. The stress lines on her face when she was at rest revealed to me some of the struggles she was enduring.

What shocked me the most was when she said doctors had removed part of her stomach. Weeks before the surgery, she was required to demonstrate the ability to lose weight by changing her eating habits. What if she had continued for a few more months? I wondered. The procedure she underwent is called bariatric surgery. The idea was to limit the amount of food she could eat in an attempt to help her lose weight. I knew that the stomach had the capacity to hold about a quart of food. That was about the size of her fist. I wasn't sure what she'd looked like right after the surgery, but it was obvious that the body fat she had lost had come right back. She worked as hard as she could during our training sessions. I knew I had to be careful with how hard I pushed her. We did body-weight exercises, boxing, and lots of dynamic stretching. Her coordination and balance were those of an athlete. Although she enjoyed our sessions, the fat didn't come off. Why? When I visited the website of the "health center" where she'd had the procedure performed, the reason was plain and clear. The pre-surgery and post-surgery diet suggestions comprised a long list of low-nutrient, pro-inflammatory foods. In other words, this facility was promoting the same pro-inflammatory foods that most likely led to her body-fat issues in the first place. Cottage cheese, ground beef, soft-boiled eggs, ground chicken, scrambled eggs, ground turkey, and fish were all listed as foods okay to eat after having a portion of your stomach removed? It may sound like malpractice, but these popular procedures are legal and performed with client consent.

Another woman who trained with me had numerous surgeries for cancerous tumors. She had the heart of a lion. We made great progress with hitting the focus mitts and other intense activities. She told me about her struggles with hot flashes and poor digestion. Her doctors removed parts of her intestines, thyroid, and entire gallbladder. She took a series of prescribed experimental chemicals. Every day she dealt with pain and discomfort. I began to further familiarize myself with the functions of these organs. The more I read, the more I could not understand why anyone would remove these body parts. Doctors I've spoken to all tell me they were taught to identify the location and stage of the visible dis-ease. She told me that none of the dozens of visits she made to her doctors addressed her lifestyle as a possible factor in her dis-ease. Instead of pinpointing the probable causes of stones in her kidneys or gallbladder, they were trained to remove the organs, like mechanics change car parts. Each and every part of the body serves a purpose. Some are beneficial in ways we don't yet fully understand. In most cases, an injured organ will heal on its own if given the necessary time and conditions.

I've met individuals who had kidneys removed to donate to family members and friends. None of these recipients were born with defects. Sacrificing a vital organ is one of the most selfless acts imaginable. These acts of bravery are commendable, but are they always necessary? I've seen how years of unhealthy living can damage organs beyond repair. Surgical intervention has saved many lives, especially when time and circumstance leave no other option. But what if these examples of organ damage were preventable or reversible without surgery? Why not educate doctors to explore other options instead? Why not inform patients about the causes of their illnesses, then guide them toward the lifestyle changes necessary to heal naturally? This way, the organ volunteer can avoid surgery and the recipient would lead by example to prevent others from suffering the same fate. The remarkable human body is often able to compensate after organs are removed. A single kidney may grow much larger in size to continue its responsibility of cleansing blood and lymph fluids. What if a damaged body was put in an environment where it was allowed to heal on its own schedule? Isn't this what all living things are designed to do?

I'm always thinking of practical ways to share valuable information with my clients. I try to accommodate their preferred methods of learning. I recommend books, send them article links, the latest evidence-based research studies, etc. Among those in the medical field, nutritional science is not promoted like it should be. One of my goals is to supply people around me with the facts. This way, they can weigh their options to make the most informed decision. A few clients followed their doctors, who convinced them that removing their dis-eased organs was the best choice. It's disappointing that they were not presented with more alternatives. I would talk to myself to try to come up with solutions. This kept me up for a few nights. One day while researching on my laptop, I came across a YouTube video that had been posted within the hour. It was made by a doctor I had spoken to several years earlier. It was all about the gallbladder, the same subject I was researching. It was so informative that I watched the ten-minute video twice. The next day while I was watching it for a third time, I received a text message. It was from the wife of one of my clients. He had been making immense improvement, but now she had taken him to the emergency room. He was experiencing severe abdominal pain, nausea, vomiting, and fever. After reviewing the CT (computer tomography) scans with the doctor, he elected to have surgery. The doctors would remove his inflamed gallbladder. I froze in disbelief when I read the text.

In most cases, gallstones are made up of cholesterol. Months earlier, we'd talked about animal products and saturated fats from oils. Judging from our previous conversations, these were the main sources of his excess cholesterol. He became more motivated to improve his eating habits. I knew he had been increasing the number of plants on his plate. I saw the improvement during our training sessions. His stamina was better. He was losing body fat. There were a few setbacks during social outings when he'd occasionally overindulge in poor food choices, but he was making tremendous progress on the whole. He was even open to going meatless on most days during the week. Among other tasks, the gallbladder stores bile from the liver. Bile is important in breaking down fat. Continuing to lower his body-fat percentage was one of our main goals for the summer. Once a vital organ was removed, keeping his body-fat percentage in a healthy range would be difficult for him.

I knew his recovery from the operation would be a lifelong challenge. It can be exponentially burdensome when we unknowingly repeat mistakes. I remained confident that he would prevent a recurrence of the gallstones by continuing to add more plants to his diet. We're communal creatures of habit. The support system around us is vital in our making and staying committed to lifestyle changes. Our bodies can never be the same once a part of the original design is removed. In an emergency situation, surgery may be the only option. We need to identify the warning signs earlier, especially if there's a pattern of a particular set of symptoms among family members. Throughout the years I've taught myself how to use the medical system's strengths to my advantage. I've also learned to identify its weaknesses and work around them. I find it impressive how well trained doctors are in diagnosis. They have access to the latest medical innovations and can accurately describe symptoms. On the flip side, none of the ones my insurance policies covered was ever trained in offering cause or cure. Unless they took it upon themselves to pursue this skill set after med school, physicians could not share natural solutions with their patients. Yearly checkups have been a great way for me to use medical expertise in diagnosis to stay ahead of any potential problems. I've learned to pay closer attention to minor details and research solutions on my own. Chronic disease is a slow process. The aches and pains along the way are teachable moments if we pay attention to what our bodies are trying to communicate. The current medical model does not teach this. Therefore, I will continue to seek information from reputable sources and educate myself as much as possible.

GEMS: I've been saddened to witness individuals consenting to questionable medical procedures, particularly the removal of organs. Consequently, I've learned to refrain from giving unsolicited advice. I'm not a medical doctor and I can feel pain or discomfort only in my own body. I listen to it and encourage others to listen to theirs. I offer moral support to friends and family in whatever capacity I can. Regrettably, there are still medical professionals who hold the belief that certain body parts, like the appendix, are vestigial and devoid of any significant function. Contrary to this misconception, compelling evidence demonstrates that the appendix serves as a reservoir for vital gut bacteria. Furthermore, some health-care practitioners remain unaware of the potential consequences, such as inflammatory bowel disease, that can arise from removing organs essential for specific bodily functions. My observations have taught me to appreciate the importance of being well versed in interpreting the latest medical studies and seeking multiple expert opinions before making a decision that could alter one's life trajectory.

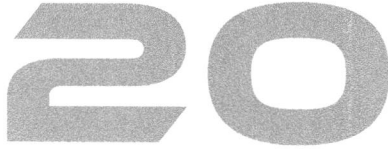

SALTY SECRETS: LESSONS ON SODIUM AND HEALTH

Excess dietary sodium promotes urinary calcium loss, leading to calcium loss from bone and therefore decreased bone density.
— Dr. Joel Fuhrman

Each of us has a body odor that is uniquely ours. Think of these odor types like another set of fingerprints. When we perspire because of heat, physical exertion, etc., our smell becomes more pronounced.

As a young man who ate lots of dead animal flesh, dairy, and processed foods, I was always worried about my body odor. I wore copious amounts of cologne to impersonate floral, earthy, and vegetative scents. After almost every meal, I was looking for breath mints, gum, or candy to disguise what I'd eaten. My mom taught me from an early age to perform the hand-to-mouth breath test. This was when you cupped one hand in front of your mouth and exhaled forcefully to catch the rebound of air off of your hand. If it smelled bad, then

I had to brush my teeth right away. If I misplaced my toothbrush, I'd reach for some mouthwash.

Most of the food I ate caused my breath to smell bad. I didn't have halitosis, but I knew something was off. The longer I went without some type of camouflage, the worse my breath smelled. Why did I continue to eat this way? Was bad breath a sign from my body to stay away from these foods? As a kid, I didn't have much of a choice. If I didn't eat what my family ate, there were no other available options. When I started earning an allowance, I would spend it mostly on pizza, vanilla ice cream, burgers, Chinese food, candy, chips, and other junk food. Why? They tasted good, these were things my friends ate, and I was addicted to the stimulation these foods gave.

As I got older, I started to pay more attention to the way my body was reacting. After graduating from college, eating out at Jamaican restaurants became a frequent practice. I would always order brown rice, peas, fish (red snapper, kingfish, or salmon), thick oxtail gravy, cabbage, and fried plantains. When I was younger, the mere sight of the head of a dead fish would've made me nauseous. Now I was eating everything but the eyeballs. I had heard that rice contained arsenic and was known to accumulate harmful heavy metals, but it remained a staple in my diet. Sometimes I'd also order a hot patty filled with cooked veggies. This was something I did at least two to three times per week. I would play pickup basketball the same number of times a week outdoors. After an hour or so of sweating profusely, I'd notice that my sweat was salty. Really salty! Whenever I'd wipe my brow, I'd rub the crystals of salt between my fingers. I'd look in the mirror and notice white streaks of salt all over my head. Something didn't seem right. My body was losing what felt like an abnormal amount of salt. Antibacterial soaps and industrial-strength antiperspirants couldn't keep my funky body odor in check. Eventually I'd stop using those products. The aluminum chloride and other chemicals in them dried my skin and caused dark armpit rashes. The body is supposed to perspire. Its odor shouldn't be offensive, though. I thought I was eating healthy foods. I made sure to include low carbs, lots of protein and fat. I'd drink around a gallon of water a day. That's what the popular bodybuilding and fitness magazines at the time said to do.

Around the same time, I woke up one morning with an unusual soreness on my back. When I tried to sit back on a chair, I was in pain. I winced each time my back made contact with the seat. I had to stand. With my back to the bathroom mirror and positioning a handheld mirror in front of me, I located a red swelling on my back the size of a golf ball. It felt like a golf ball. I was nervous. What the hell was it? A trip to a dermatologist revealed that it was a boil. I'd never had that before.

"What causes a boil?" I asked, visibly nervous.

"They're quite common. When I was a teenager, I used to get them," she replied in an East Indian accent.

I rephrased the question. "Where do boils come from?"

"It's a bacterial infection that usually goes away with medicine. It's no big deal."

"Was it something that I did?"

"Does anyone else in your family have them?"

"Not that I know of."

"Then, I wouldn't worry about it. I will give you a cream that will make it disappear in a week or two."

I could not get her to give me a straight answer. As expected, I was given a prescription for some steroid cream to use daily until the boil disappeared. After about a week, the swelling subsided. This was nice, but I still wanted answers. There was important information I wasn't getting. I had to find it.

I began researching the role diet and family medical history play in health. Diabetes and arthritis were no strangers to my mom's side of the family. Heart and prostate issues were a few that ran rampant on my father's side. I read that poor nutrition is one of the leading risk factors that make us susceptible to dis-ease. The boil on my back was my body attempting to communicate with me. My lymphatic system, aka waste-management system, was trying to deal with an accumulation of toxins. The boil was the process of inflammation progressing into the later stages of dis-ease. The red swelling and pain were the results of blood being directed by an immune response to heal. The pro-inflammatory foods we ate were the main causes of dis-ease on my maternal and paternal sides of the family. With wisdom comes responsibility. I began to focus on how I could replace these foods with healthier options.

There's Sodium and Then There's Salt

The Food and Drug Administration reported that the average American in 2020–2021 consumed more than 3,400 milligrams of salt per day. The FDA recommended less than a teaspoon, or 2,300 milligrams per day. In 2010, the U.S. Dietary Guidelines set the recommended daily level of salt intake at 1,500 milligrams for African Americans, people older than age fifty, and individuals with diabetes, chronic kidney dis-ease, or elevated blood pressure. Fifteen hundred milligrams is equal to three quarters of a teaspoon. It was tough to tell exactly how much was in the restaurant food I was eating. I knew it was way too much. With the abundance of fast-food restaurants in African American neighborhoods, salt levels are almost always on overload. Yes, too much of anything can be bad, but what is it about salt? I had plenty of questions.

I read anything I could find about dietary salt and how our bodies respond to it. Articles on the internet allowed me to better understand how salt is an abusive irritant to human tissue. The real-life applications became obvious. The examples that were hidden in plain sight finally began to make sense to me. Why do we feel a burning sensation when salt is poured over an open wound? Ever see a slug or snail react to salt granules on its moist skin? It quickly becomes dehydrated. It flinches and squirms in agony. I remember all the times I swam in salt water and the water accidentally went in my mouth. Why did I feel so dehydrated each and every time I came out the water? What about all those trips to the beach when I had salt water go up my nose? Why did the salt water irritate the sinus membrane and cause a burning sensation? Why did blood rush to protect my eyes whenever they were exposed to salt water? Why does drinking a concentrated salt solution make me want to vomit and get it out of my system as quickly as possible? If 70 percent of the Earth's surface is covered in salt water, why are we increasingly facing extreme water shortages? I have never seen bottled ocean water for sale. What made me think that salt extracted from the seas and oceans was somehow now a health food? Desalination, or removing salt from seawater for human consumption, will be a common practice for decades to come.

I discovered that salt serves no nutritional benefit in my body. Yes. You read that correctly. I found out through trial and error that salt is not compatible with my digestive system. But wait. Isn't sodium an electrolyte? Wouldn't I need it for my muscles to contract and for the proper transmission of nerve impulses? Wouldn't sodium help control my blood pressure and blood volume? What about chloride? Doesn't chloride help regulate fluids in the human body and assist in digestion? Wouldn't a lack of dietary chloride lead to muscle weakness, loss of appetite, and lethargy? Yes, sodium and chloride are essential for my body to thrive, but not all salt is the same.

The words *sodium* and *salt* are often used interchangeably, but their chemical makeups can be quite different. They occur naturally but because their chemical structures are not the same, my body treated some favorably and the others unfavorably. Sodium (Na) in its organic form is an essential element for all animals. It can be found in whole plants. Then, there is salt

(NaCl), aka sodium chloride, which I have unknowingly been overexposed to for most of my life. These salts can be harmful and have promoted dis-ease in my body.

Organic sodium (Na)—Healthy	Inorganic salts (NaCl)—Not a Health Food
Celery—30 mg per stalk	Sea salts
Chard—179 mg per 100 g	Table salt
Spinach—24 mg per cup	Pink salt
Seaweeds	Alaea salt
Beets—120 mg per cup	Kosher salt
Fruits & vegetables	Processed foods

What do I mean? Sodium or salt in its organic form is what my body needs. No, I'm not talking about a certified organic label on a food package, in a health food store, or in a supermarket section. I'm referring to the chemical makeup of sodium that existed long before corporations decided to monetize the term *organic*. The organic sodium I'm referring to is found naturally in living plant foods. How? Here's an example. Dolomite is a mineral found in limestone. I'd surely break my teeth if I tried to eat such a hard rock. However, through microbial activity, organic matter decomposition, and organic acids from plant roots, dolomite slowly dissolves and releases calcium and magnesium ions into the soil environment. Plants are then able to absorb these essential calcium ions through their root systems. Photosynthesis allows plants to incorporate the calcium from dissolved dolomite into their plant tissues and structures. Now, that's something I can sink my teeth into. The best source of calcium and other minerals I need in order to thrive comes from plants. Only plants can transform inorganic minerals from the earth and water into organic minerals that my body can use to help me live my best life. Plants need calcium to keep their cell walls and structure intact. I need the calcium in plants to help keep my skeletal system and structure complete. Iodine is another element I found out was essential for human health. Trace amounts are included in some iodized salts. Globally, two billion people lack the dietary iodine necessary for proper brain, heart, and thyroid function. It has even been known to assist in removing fluoride from the pineal gland. I began to search for plants like nori, kelp, and other seaweeds to provide safer sources of iodine.

Then there's the other salt. The salt that is now commonly used in cooked and processed food (table salt, sea salt, bamboo salt, etc.) is sodium chloride. Sodium chloride is salt in its inorganic form. In other words, it does not come from living matter. I discovered that my body has an unfavorable response to salt not derived from living matter. In nature, sodium chloride is an ionic compound, or a bond: a bond that my body desperately tries to break apart with water whenever I consume sodium chloride. Why? Because my body's wisdom knows that it's just a matter of time before the sodium chloride causes destruction. That's why eating salty meals or snacks instantly gives me a dry mouth and makes me thirsty. My brain sends an SOS signal, telling me to consume more water immediately. When I drink water, the blood carries the water into the tissue fluids to dilute the harmful effects of the sodium chloride. Shortly after ingesting sodium chloride, I wouldn't urinate for hours—normally, I'd pass urine eight to twelve times per day. When I finally did, it was much darker and more pungent than usual. My body had concentrated the salt to remove as much of it as possible. I noticed that whenever overweight or obese personal training clients of mine got on board to eat more produce, I detected a pattern. Sometimes I'd have them consult a handheld body fat–loss monitor. The first pounds that came off were mostly water weight. Their bodies had been holding on to water in attempts to dilute the excess inorganic salt they had been eating. Because less inorganic salt was now coming in, their bodies felt comfortable enough to let go of the excess water.

Not to be confused with sodium chloride, sodium and chloride individually are two highly beneficial elements. Minimally processed ripe fruits, vegetables, nuts, seeds, and various sprouts contain the best sources of sodium and chloride in abundance. Whole plants naturally present these elements in a recognizable molecular structure that my body can use for proper cell function, lymphatic system maintenance, and other vital functions, some of which were mentioned earlier.

Sodium chloride did not dissolve in my body like I'd originally thought. Instead, it was stored in my body and was excreted by my body as sodium chloride. That's why it appeared on my skin in its original crystal-like chemical form. The two elements remained bonded. My body used perspiration to try to remove it as quickly as possible. Sodium chloride irritated and destroyed my cells, membranes, and tissues from the moment it entered my body until the time it was excreted.

Other articles I read went on to describe how salt (sodium chloride) negatively affects the body's cells, causing them to discharge their life fluids, thus leading to heart defects, high blood pressure, muscle cramps, blindness, ulcers, tumors, hardened arteries, destruction to the interior lining of blood vessels, and disruption of balance in the gut microbiome. I can still remember waking up with leg-muscle cramps in the middle of the night when I was in high school. It's a sudden violent pain that takes your breath away. The more I consciously cut back on inorganic salt over the years, the fewer cramps I experienced. I've known people who shook the saltshaker over every meal. It became a reflex reaction. They'd reach for the salt before they had any idea of what the food tasted like. To the untrained eye, they may have appeared unblemished, but internally, we all have various processes that occur simultaneously at different speeds.

The new information I was seeking sounded like I was reading the Gospel. Sodium chloride is an anti-biotic. *Anti* means against. *Bio* means life. It's commonly known to have been used as a preservative to kill bacteria or life for many years. It prevents the natural decomposition of dead organisms. Just one ounce is enough to kill a human. I, like many other people, argued that salt added "taste" to enhance the flavor of food. I tried putting some salt on the tip of my finger. It had no taste. How can something that has no taste add flavor to my food? In actuality, it numbs the salt taste receptors on my tongue.

So, what's the verdict? A wide variety of fresh, living plants provide all the essential sodium I need. These foods contain the best sodium in the right amounts, allowing me to reach my daily caloric requirements with no concern of overdosing. On the other hand, my body treated processed, nonplant salts like addictive drugs, stimulating the pleasure-seeking hormone (dopamine) in my brain, tempting me to eat more of it. I didn't realize how much salt I had been consuming over the years. My introduction to sodium chloride probably went as far back as store-bought baby food. If it passed my parents' taste test, they then fed it to me. That's where it begins for everyone. From then on, the more inorganic salt I consumed, the more challenging it was to endure the withdrawal symptoms whenever I tried to reduce or eliminate its intake. My father suffered an ischemic stroke when he was in his early seventies. A blocked artery limited the blood flow to his brain. He never fully recovered. Through my studies, I learned that salt consumption increased the likelihood of hemorrhagic stroke. This type of stroke results in bleeding in and around the brain. I didn't want to suffer either type of stroke. That was a major motivator in my cutting back my salt intake more each year. When transitioning from a high-salt diet, eating plants without added salt can seem like eating tasteless leaves because their sodium content is so low in comparison. It took time to recondition my taste buds to appreciate the milder flavors that nature has to offer. It was like watching a classic movie shot in black and white and learning to find value in the art of fine acting. More modern multimillion-dollar budgets, explosions, and immersive technologies can provide entertainment while distracting an audience from a poorly written script, below par postproduction, and/or an inexperienced cast and crew. I was fixated on artificial flavors, when the more important aspect of food to focus on is micronutrients. These nutrients are required in trace amounts and are vital for normal growth and development. Remove all the commercial hype from heavily marketed foods and you're left with a low-quality product at its core. Salt was a major factor in making poor food choices palatable for many years.

I noticed that when I stuck to a mostly raw regimen of fresh produce, outdoor activities in the hot sun were easier. Whenever I played basketball, ran miles, or performed calisthenics, I no longer saw the white streaks of salt on my skin. I barely drank a half gallon of water a day and was not thirsty after hours of exercise outdoors. I had more energy for longer periods of time. My body was better able to utilize and maintain the sodium in its organic form.

Coming off of an artificially stimulating diet of salty, nutritionally void foods can offer a variety of challenges. The perception of enhanced taste and minimized bitterness are some of the most common. This perceived heightened flavor actually came from my sense of smell. Salt is added in almost every food these days. Salt content is the first thing I look for whenever I pick up a package with a nutritional label. I've found it best to avoid foods with labels, but if I choose not to, I'll use a magnifying glass app on my phone. I've noticed a dramatic decrease in font size over the years . . . hmm. Even if I have no plans on purchasing the item, I'm still amazed at the high amounts put into popular packaged foods. Many restaurants have nutrition calculators. Whenever possible, I try to research menu ingredients before eating out. The salt amounts in modern-day refined foods are astounding. Some restaurant chains have entrées with 2,500 mg minimums and patrons continue to fill these eateries to capacity every week! Buyer beware.

I'm still a work in progress. On days when I consume completely raw fruits, vegetables, nuts, and /or seeds, my organic sodium intake is around 600 to 700 mg. That satisfies my needs. The organic salt and its surrounding components eliminate bloating, poor digestion, low energy, and all the other issues that inorganic salt consumption caused me. In my experience, consuming the recommended 1,500 mg per day of salt would still be noticeably harmful. Staying far below that number is ideal for me. I don't feel the need to take potassium chloride, magnesium chloride, or other salts, either, because I easily get them from produce. I haven't reached an intake of 100 percent raw produce every day. Most people living in an industrialized society won't have, either. I simply keep refined-salt consumption as low as possible. Substituting salt with seasonings and spices have helped me to curve cravings tremendously.

Organic paprika, oregano, onion powder, cinnamon, garlic powder, dulse, kelp flakes, dill, and nutritional yeast are some of my favorites to add to salads and soups. Celery, olives, tomatoes, and lettuce are great sources of chloride and some of the highest natural sodium foods for electrolyte balance. As harmful as sodium chloride has been to me, my body allowed me to take in higher amounts over time. Why? In order to keep me alive. I haven't heard of too many people dying after smoking their first cigarette, drinking their first glass of alcohol, or eating their first double cheeseburger. There may be coughing, vomiting, or other violent reactions to these harmful substances the first time. It's a shock to the body's systems. In order to preserve life, the body may gradually allow for more toxic consumption. Over time, a person may graduate to smoking a pack of cigarettes a day, drinking a full bottle of alcohol, or competing in an eating contest. Eventually, the organs of elimination (skin, kidneys, liver) will prematurely break down and the body will choose when and how to stop the destruction. Having said that, I notice the positive differences when cutting back on cooked foods for days, weeks, even months at a time. Living produce has improved my skin clarity, athletic performance, digestive regularity, and keeps me feeling hydrated even on the hottest days. I'm happy with how my body odor has transformed. I haven't worn cologne or chewed gum in decades. These days I opt for natural soaps and deodorants with the least number of chemical ingredients. Inflammation has decreased, and overall, my health has gotten noticeably better.

GEMS: Roughly 60 to 70 percent of the human body is water. It's no coincidence that most fruits and vegetables contain at least 70 percent water. I realized that eating foods below that percentage of water dehydrated me. An easier way to keep skin looking younger is to hydrate by eating water-rich foods. Dr. Gerald Pollack, author of *The Fourth Phase of Water: Beyond Solid, Liquid, and Vapor,* is credited with discovering a fourth phase of water found in plant and human cells. When water comes in contact with our cells, it becomes EZ (exclusion zone) water, or H_3O_2, a highly structured, gel-like water charged by electrolytes. This living water is more alkaline. It can hold energy from the sun like a battery and deliver it in ways regular water can't. Urinating at least several times each day has been a positive sign of health for me. As an athlete, light yellow urine has been an accurate indicator of good hydration. The more calories that come from live, mineral-rich fruits and vegetables, the better I feel my chances are of staying healthy. I've been able to solve previous dehydration issues by consuming more water.

21

SHOPPING CARTS FULL OF SYMPTOMS: HIDDEN IN PLAIN SIGHT

Water and air, the two essential fluids on which all life depends, have become global garbage cans.
— Jacques Cousteau

March 2020. Living in the United States for any significant amount of time means you probably know someone who has been affected by heart disease, cancer, or stroke. As a self-proclaimed social scientist, I was always frustrated by how little I understood about these debilitating conditions. That is until a routine exchange of office emails with my colleagues opened my eyes to a startling reality.

Every month, one of my coworkers would share a collection of photos featuring the most unusual characters shopping at Walmart stores across the country. What struck me was that a majority of these unwitting subjects were either morbidly obese or overweight, a snapshot of the alarming statistics I had read about the average American. Some wore clothing that was clearly too small, while others appeared to have simply rolled out of bed and made their way to the nearest location in whatever they had on. As my colleagues and I chuckled at the absurdity of some of the images, I couldn't help but recognize the serious underlying issues these individuals were grappling with.

Walking through the fluorescent-lit aisles of Walmart, I felt like a curious anthropologist observing the rituals of the average American consumer. The store was a sprawling labyrinth of wide aisles and towering shelves, filled with everything from discount electronics to bulk bags of potato chips. It was a mecca for those seeking convenience and affordability, a place where the allure of a bargain was hard to resist.

But as I made my way through the food section, I couldn't help but be struck by the display reflecting the average American's shopping habits. The shelves were stocked with highly processed, calorie-dense foods, marketed with bright colors and catchy slogans. It was a dizzying array of choices, and I found it utterly fascinating.

As I walked past row after row of sugary cereals, snack cakes, and frozen dinners, I couldn't help but wonder how many people had been lured into these unhealthy choices. Was it the convenience of prepackaged meals? The appeal of a quick sugar rush? Or simply a lack of awareness about the impact of these foods on their health?

For me, the Walmart experience was a wake-up call. It made me realize just how important it is to be mindful of what we put into our bodies. By making a conscious effort to choose whole, nutrient-dense foods, we can improve our physical health, mental clarity, and overall well-being.

It wasn't long before I found myself becoming a Walmart shopper myself. The convenience and affordability of the store's offerings were undeniable, and it seemed like new locations were popping up everywhere. But as I pushed my cart through the aisles, I couldn't help but wonder if the people I had seen in those emails from my coworkers were real. Were the morbidly obese and overweight individuals I had laughed at in those pictures actually shopping here?

As someone who had been on my own journey toward better health, I was acutely aware of the impact of nutrition on our bodies. I had spent countless hours researching the science of nutrition to understand how our food choices affect our health. And what I saw in the shopping carts of many of the Walmart patrons left me with a sense of disbelief.

The aisles were filled with packaged dead animals, dairy products, breads, cookies, crackers, pastas, cakes, sugary drinks, and various processed foods. Tobacco and alcohol also seemed to be popular items that were often purchased at the checkout line with proper identification. Occasionally, I would spot an obese person in the produce section, picking up a few bananas or a bag of potatoes or apples. But never once did I see an obese person with a shopping cart or basket full of produce. Not even after countless trips to Walmarts across different states in this country.

It was a stark contrast to what I had learned about nutrition and its importance in maintaining a healthy lifestyle. Popular media often blamed obesity on hereditary factors, or "fat genes," but my observations told a different story. The largest, most overweight individuals I had ever seen seemed to frequent these stores, filling their carts with highly processed, sugary, and unhealthy foods.

I couldn't help but wonder how these individuals had accumulated so many pounds of body fat. Was it truly just genetics, or was there something else at play? The disconnect between what I had learned about nutrition and what I was observing regarding the shopping habits of many Americans was baffling. It was a puzzle that I was determined to unravel, and it fueled my curiosity to dig deeper into the root causes of poor health and obesity.

As I pushed my cart through the aisles, I felt a sense of urgency to continue my research, a process of self-discovery through trial and error in my pursuit of better health. The aisles of Walmart became a reminder of the need for education, awareness, and a shift in our food culture. I knew that I had a role to play in spreading knowledge and making a difference, not just for myself but for others who were struggling with their health, as well.

With each trip to Walmart, I was increasingly motivated to share my findings, challenge the status quo, and inspire change. The journey toward better health was not just about my own well-being but about the well-being of our society as a whole.

In 2020, as the world went into lockdown, social interactions became a distant memory. It was as if we were all kids again, being scolded by authority figures and told that we couldn't play with our friends or see our family members in person. The impact of this isolation was palpable, affecting the physical and mental well-being of both young and old alike. It was all too easy to succumb to the temptation of staying indoors, neglecting self-care, and losing touch with reality.

Forced to confront our true selves, stripped of the usual masks we wore—outfits, makeup, and social personas—many of us found solace in solitude. Personally, I had always been comfortable being alone, and this period presented a unique opportunity for more self-discovery. But as I ventured out, I couldn't ignore the palpable anxiety, fear, and despair that hung in the air. Even though masks and face wraps concealed our identities, the pain was unmistakable in people's eyes. The online purchases of tobacco and alcohol skyrocketed, a clear sign that the effects of depression and other mental health issues were taking hold of those around me.

It was a sobering realization that while the physical health risks of the lockdown were widely discussed, the toll it was taking on our mental well-being was equally significant. The once vibrant and bustling streets now echoed with emptiness, and the absence of human connection left a void that couldn't be filled by material possessions or virtual interactions. We were all craving the warmth of a hug, the comfort of a shared meal, and the laughter of loved ones. Yet these simple pleasures seemed like distant dreams, a luxury we couldn't afford in the midst of a global crisis.

But amid the darkness, there was a glimmer of hope. I realized that this period of isolation was a wake-up call, urging us to prioritize our health, both physical and mental. It was a reminder to peel off the layers of societal expectations and delve into the depths of our souls. It was an invitation to confront our fears, anxieties, and insecurities head-on, and emerge stronger.

As I navigated through the challenges of the lockdown, I learned the importance of self-care, not just physically but emotionally and mentally, as well. I discovered new ways to connect with others, even from a distance—through virtual conversations, shared hobbies, and acts of kindness. I found solace in nature, immersing myself in the healing power of the outdoors. I sought refuge in creativity, indulging in art, music, and literature as an escape from the bleak reality of daily life.

It wasn't easy, and there were moments when the weight of the situation felt overwhelming. But I realized that I was not alone. Countless others were facing similar struggles, and we were all in this together. We were learning, adapting, and growing, despite the challenges that were thrown our way.

In the midst of the chaos, I found a renewed sense of purpose—to prioritize my health and well-being, to cherish the value of human connection, and never to take the simple joys of life for granted. The lockdown may have forced us to wear masks, but it also stripped away the masks we had been wearing all along, revealing our true selves and reminding us of what truly matters.

As the world slowly emerged from the grips of the lockdown, I realized that I had come out of it a changed person. I had gained a deeper understanding of myself, developed new coping mechanisms, and learned the importance of resilience in the face of adversity.

I also understood I had the power to control my own behavior and influence my well-being. One of the first changes I made was in my morning routine. I learned that the words and images I exposed myself to upon waking could set the tone for the entire day. So I made it a habit to limit the amount of news and other media I consumed in the morning.

The legacy media thrives on sensationalism, and I noticed that flowers blossoming and birds chirping in nature didn't make for the type of ratings they were looking for. Instead, it was the negative narratives and fear-inducing stories that dominated the headlines. I realized that by embracing positive words and limiting my exposure to negative media, I could create a more uplifting and empowering start to my day.

Just like how I consumed water to nourish my body, I realized that the words I consumed also had a profound impact on my mental and emotional well-being. I became more conscious of the language I used with myself and others, and I made a conscious effort to surround myself with positivity. I learned that the words we speak and the stories we tell ourselves shape our reality, and I became more intentional about choosing empowering narratives that supported my health and well-being.

I couldn't help but marvel at the incredible complexity and resilience of the human body. I've never known life on Earth without bacteria, germs, viruses, etc. I realized that our immune function plays a starring role in protecting us against premature death. It had been a constant companion since the day I was born, silently working to keep me healthy and alive. I also observed that in nature, it is often the weakest animals that are the first to fall prey to illness and disease. It made me realize the importance of taking care of my physical health, and I made conscious efforts to nourish my body with healthy foods, regular exercise, and meaningful interactions with others.

One thing that struck me was the prevalence of obesity and unhealthy habits in our society. I realized that it was not a characteristic of those who lived the longest among us. In fact, the daily habits that led to an unhealthy state seemed to be a pandemic that had been going on long before 2020. I couldn't help but notice that these behaviors were barely addressed by the authorities with the most influence and power over the masses. It made me question the societal norms and expectations around health and wellness, and I became more determined to make conscious choices that supported my own well-being.

As I navigated through public spaces, I didn't measure the distance I kept from others. I didn't have to. I could always sense if I was invading someone's personal space, and vice versa. It was common sense to keep a distance from someone who was coughing, sneezing, or showing obvious symptoms of illness. However, I couldn't help but question the notion that staying an exact distance away from an infected person would prevent disease from spreading. It seemed overly simplistic and unrealistic to me. I realized that there were many factors at play when it came to the spread of disease, and it required a more nuanced approach, one that took into consideration the complexity of human behavior and the environment.

I had come to realize that true well-being goes beyond just physical health. It is a holistic approach that encompasses our mental, emotional, and social well-being also. It requires a deeper understanding of ourselves and our environment, and a willingness to question conventional wisdom and embrace a more empowered and intentional way of living.

Years ago, I stumbled upon the works of Antoine Béchamp, a French biologist who had been a proponent of the terrain theory back in the 1800s. This groundbreaking theory argued that the environment of the gut, where the majority of our body's immunity resides, plays a pivotal role in determining the likelihood of disease. It made perfect sense to me that an unhealthy gut environment would be a breeding ground for dis-ease. It was clear that a healthy lifestyle, including a plant-exclusive nutrition plan, could foster a robust gut microbiome that would be better equipped to defend against disease.

Béchamp was known not only for his pioneering theories but also for his fierce rivalry with Louis Pasteur, a prominent chemist and microbiologist who championed the germ theory. According to Pasteur's theory, microorganisms or pathogens invade the human body and reproduce, causing disease. However, despite Béchamp's groundbreaking research, the medical community had largely dismissed his terrain theory and embraced Pasteur's germ theory as the prevailing explanation for disease.

As I continued to navigate locked-down areas, I couldn't help but observe the stark contradictions in how society was responding to the crisis. At the height of the lockdown, there were long lines outside stores, and social distancing reminders were plastered everywhere in the form of stickers and signs. Self-checkout counters had employees diligently sanitizing touch screens, shopping carts, and baskets after each use. But this heightened sense of caution seemed to dissipate after a month or two, and soon enough, I noticed that hands were once again touching dirty screens, doors, baskets, and shopping carts with reckless abandon.

What saddened me even more was that little had changed in the Western diet and lifestyle, which had long been identified as a major contributor to dis-ease. Despite the overwhelming evidence linking poor lifestyle choices to various health issues, including those that worsened the impact of the crisis, there seemed to be little emphasis on adopting healthier habits. Instead, city and state officials were promoting beer, doughnuts, and fried chicken as incentives for getting experimental chemical injections, with some drug manufacturers even hinting at the possibility of additional booster shots in the future.

I couldn't believe my eyes when I saw a video of New York City mayor Bill de Blasio sitting at a press conference, enthusiastically urging New Yorkers to get vaccinated while simultaneously munching on a greasy hamburger and French fries. It was ironic, to say the least. Weren't these the very foods that contributed to the preexisting conditions that had made so many people vulnerable to getting sick in the first place? The CDC had admitted that nearly 80 percent of COVID-19 hospitalizations were among individuals who were overweight or obese, and heart disease had claimed twice as many lives in 2020. The link between poor lifestyle choices and health issues had been established for decades. It seemed absurd to me that junk foods, laden with unhealthy fats and empty calories, were being offered as incentives, while nutrient-rich fruits and vegetables were largely ignored.

I couldn't help but wonder why a preventive approach, focusing on promoting a healthy lifestyle and proper nutrition, was not being offered to those in need. It saddened me to see that amid the chaos of a crisis, the opportunity to prioritize long-term health and well-being had been missed. As I reflected on the works of Béchamp and his terrain theory, it became even clearer to me that building a strong foundation of health through a plant-exclusive nutrition plan and an active lifestyle was the key not only to slowing down aging but also improving overall well-being.

As I step outside now, I'm struck by the sight of people with their faces covered, even when they're alone in their cars or outdoors in wide-open spaces. It's been years since the restrictions were lifted nationwide and around the world, but the trauma of the past events still lingers for many. I remember the fear that gripped so many, the health scares and the heartbreak of losing loved ones to illness. And while some found solace in staying indoors, shielding themselves from adversity, the impact of reentering society under different terms has left a significant portion of the population permanently shaken.

The ability to cope with increased challenges is not a skill possessed by the masses. We've become more sensitive, more insecure. The global events of 2020 were a missed opportunity, a moment for the world to wake up, to reject confirmation bias and unlearn false theories. It was a chance to embrace proven scientific facts, to learn from the consequences of our unhealthy habits. But instead, psychological fear tactics perpetuated an unproven germ theory, keeping the masses masked and anticipating the next variant.

As I look ahead, I can't help but feel a sense of foreboding. The polar ices continue to melt, water levels rise, and floods ravage coastlines. Fires rage unchecked, the Earth shakes with increasing violence, and species after species of insects and animals slip into extinction. Clean water, once taken for granted, becomes scarcer by the day. It's a harsh reality, a consequence of man's relentless destruction of nature. And with each passing day, a new variant, as always, looms on the horizon, a consequence of our shortsightedness and disregard for the delicate balance of our planet.

But what's perhaps most disheartening is the blatant profiteering of companies that have made billions by peddling experimental chemical doses as the solution to all health woes. They've even targeted children, exploiting the fears and vulnerabilities of the masses. Meanwhile, voices that dare to question the popular germ theory are silenced, censored from the mainstream, as trendy social media platforms remove posts and shut down pages of influencers with dissenting opinions.

I've seen people who've retreated from society, who no longer interact with the world as they used to. Separation from society at large may have its benefits from time to time, but separating from nature is not the answer. The global populations who tend to age gracefully do not live in isolation. The fear that keeps us indoors, afraid to breathe the air or smile at other humans without face coverings, has led to serious mental disorders, especially among the young and the elderly. It's a paradox: For all the polluted air that now circulates around the globe, it's still crucial for us to seek out the best air we can and connect with our fellow beings.

As I continue my search for proven methods to prevent premature aging and improve health, I'm reminded that our well-being is intricately tied to the well-being of our planet. It's time to break free from the shackles of fear and embrace a holistic approach to health, one that encompasses not just our bodies but also our environment. It's time to unlearn the false theories that hold us back and relearn the wisdom of nature. The road ahead may be challenging, but it's a journey worth taking. For only when we truly understand our interconnectedness with the world around us can we hope to thrive, to age gracefully, and to live our lives to the fullest.

On Haitian Flag Day in 2020, my family and I laid my father's body to rest. He had battled the complications of a stroke for over a dozen years. As I stood beside his grave, I couldn't help but feel a sense of emptiness. Out of his several children, I was the only child he had with my mother, the woman he chose to be his wife. I was the only one who lived with him until adulthood. It was as if a part of me had been buried along with him. But then something clicked inside of me, and I found myself saving pineapple crowns and planting them in pots and in the ground. And before I knew it, a dozen pineapple plants had sprouted.

My newfound passion for gardening didn't stop there. I made frequent trips to local nurseries, stocking up on soil, fertilizers, minerals, bamboo staffs, and small vegetable plants. Soon enough, my yard was bursting with Everglades tomatoes, tree collards, Okinawa spinach, Cuban oregano, dragon fruit, collard greens, Russian kale, and longevity spinach.

At first, I couldn't understand why I was spending so much time and energy with my hands in the soil. But then it hit me: Gardening was one of the most intimate activities I had shared with my father. Whenever we hit the garden, his energy became calmer, more centered. And now, as I planted and nurtured life, I felt as though I was somehow connected to him still.

It gave me a rush. But not like any I had ever experienced. This was more of a euphoric nostalgia. Plants were teeming with life— from the brilliant colors, scents, and textures of nature to the potent anti-inflammatory and antiaging properties of anthocyanins, the pigments responsible for the purple, blue, and red hues of some plants. Studies had proven that anthocyanins also possess antiobesity effects and can even improve vision.

I watched in awe as my purple longevity spinach grew like weeds during the rainy season, thanks to the abundance of oxygen and vital minerals in the rainwater. I had to harvest it almost every day just to keep it from taking over the yard. But the difference it made to my health was undeniable. The anthocyanins in the spinach, blueberries, peppers, and other plants I was consuming were working in my favor.

Gardening became a therapy of sorts for me. It engaged my senses and gave me a rush of accomplishment every time I harvested a fresh crop. And solving the puzzles of proper plant interactions was both fun and challenging. It allowed me to visualize the skills and resources necessary to raise healthy children someday.

Sure, some people might warn against getting too dirty in the soil, but for me, it was worth it. Gardening worked as a great stress reliever—an activity that commanded my attention without being overdemanding. And most important, it allowed me to focus on life, to connect with my father's memory, and to nourish my body and soul.

GEMS: Sprouting with rainwater. Broccoli sprouts are some of my favorite greens to grow. Sprouts are among the most nutrient-dense foods on the planet. You don't need soil, and they'll grow almost anywhere. I'll put a tablespoon or two of certified organic sprouting seeds in a mason jar with a stainless-steel sprouting lid screen. If the forecast calls for rain, I'll place the jar outside to catch as much rain as possible and let the seeds soak for twelve hours. Rainwater is richer in oxygen and other beneficial nutrients. Rinse two or more times daily with as much rainwater as you have access to. If not, bottled water works well, too. Within two to four days, you'll have sprouts to eat. Great for salads, smoothies, sandwiches, etc.

In writing this book, I set out on a journey to share proven methods to prevent premature aging and improve health. As I've learned more about this lifestyle, I realized that growing food was not just a hobby but a necessity for the future of this planet. Food scarcity is a serious issue affecting billions of people worldwide, and the wealthy few controlling the majority of fertile farmland only exacerbates the problem. This commercial farming industry relies heavily on harmful chemicals that not only impact the quality of the food but also have detrimental effects on physical and mental health. I'm constantly learning how to improve my relationship with plants on this planet to ensure my survival, and that of future generations.

As I connected more with nature, I discovered that I share similar qualities with plants. When I'm in the right environment, I thrive, just like they do. But when I'm surrounded by negativity, I suffer, just like plants that do not receive enough sunlight or water. The common cycles of working long hours in unfulfilling jobs, enduring daily commutes, and unsatisfying relationships lead to unhappiness, which can shorten life spans.

Living a fulfilling life means standing out from the crowd and making a positive impact on the world. It is easy to conform to societal norms and blend in with everyone else, but this will not lead to a life of joy and satisfaction. If my actions are contributing to the destruction of our planet, it doesn't matter how young or healthy I may look. I've learned to take responsibility for my impact on the environment and work to create a better world for future generations.

I have come to realize that we have much more control over our health than we've been led to believe. Environment and lifestyle play a much larger role in the proliferation of disease than hereditary factors. Unfortunately, the false narratives perpetuated by powerful industries often overlook these crucial factors. In this memoir, I hope to inspire readers to rediscover nature, improve their relationship with plants, and take control of their health. These actions will enhance our environment. The time to act is now.

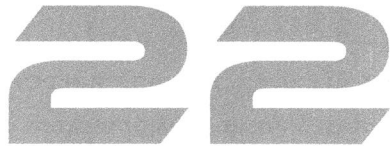

AGING GRACEFULLY: EMBRACING THE TAPESTRY OF LIFE'S JOURNEY

Once a man, twice a child.
— *Anonymous*

Back in middle school, I was envious of the kids who were a grade or two ahead of me. Whenever they challenged me to a footrace on the playground, I always came in second place. They made it look like they had the middle school routine down to a science. Some got working papers that allowed them to take part-time jobs and make extra money. I wanted the latest sneakers, jeans, and jackets, too. Graduation came and they were off to high school. When it was my turn to play freshman, I tried to mimic the upperclassmen. They experienced these amazing growth spurts during summer break. In the fall, they came back inches taller and pounds heavier. Their voices got deeper. Some kids were able to grow full beards. I got excited the first day I looked in the mirror and spotted some peach fuzz sprouting from my chin. The artist in me took creative license as far as I could. I used a black crayon to darken my mustache for more of a five o'clock shadow. I also drew in a darker goatee. The older boys made puberty look easy. They got to date the senior girls and drive them around in fancy cars. There was a huge buildup to high school graduation. The graduates were called "young adults." A few got scholarships and were about to travel out of state to attend major universities. When I got to college, I became a rebel. It was the first time I could live on my own terms. I made tons of reckless decisions. Somehow, I survived to write about them. I counted the days until I would turn twenty-one. I could legally drink in most states because I was officially an adult. Since it was no longer illegal, drinking wasn't as fun as it used to be. But my binge drinking outings were legendary. I looked forward to turning twenty-five. That was when I'd be able to rent a car with a credit card that had my name on it. Cross-country road trips looked like an incredible time in all the movies we enjoyed when we were high. I partied at nightclubs across the country. Then something happened. Shortly after turning twenty-five, I stopped hoping I'd keep getting older. I heard people say that's when the human brain goes through significant changes. When I'd been asked my age years before, I'd added a half year to whatever age I actually was. Now I was hesitant to say. I even tried to deflect my exact age and say that I was in my twenties. I was in no hurry to accomplish all the future milestones adults my age were being judged by. College graduation, getting a good paying job, marriage, children, buying a house, retirement, and death were set up as a path for me to follow. At least those were the goals that classroom conditioning, family, and pop culture taught me to pursue. I wasn't inspired to do any of those things. At least not yet.

I wanted to stay young. Not as in remaining a child, but maintaining the imagination and freedom to dream. The desire to explore without limitations and restrictions was lost among people of adult age. The curiosity and wonder they'd once possessed had been replaced by the sunken stares of rat-race conformity. I asked myself a few times if there was something off with my way of thinking. I've met only a few who seemed content in completing the common adult checklist. But I chose to defer until there was a genuine desire to devote myself selflessly to something. Maybe I was afraid of taking on serious responsibilities. Playing was important in my childhood development. It was an effective form of learning through unscripted experiences. I wanted to enjoy constructive entertainment no matter what my chronological age was. I didn't feel comfortable walking the plank that greater society laid out for adults to walk through life. It was too narrow for me. It felt more like an assembly line. A stripe that led to the end of a short, steep cliff.

I have few regrets about going to college. At first, I didn't have much of a choice. I promised my parents I would attend right after high school. In my mind, it was a show of appreciation for all they'd invested in me. Eventually I obtained a four-year degree because I like to complete whatever I start. The people I associated with, the friendships that endured, and the "education" is all a part of who I am. It was an English professor who told me during my first university semester that I had a gift to influence people with the written word. That was during a time when writing couldn't have been any lower on my list of priorities. The thousands spent on student loan principal and interest could have easily purchased Nike stocks. That was the only athletic gear I wore on campus. Share prices have exponentially increased since then. Maybe that's one of the few regrets I've learned to live with. Either way, those lessons are priceless. Constantly following a course of study was a habit that college taught me. One of the fastest ways to get old is to stop learning. As I'm writing this, my physical abilities haven't declined. In fact, I'm able to do things athletically that a younger version of myself could only have dreamed of. I still enjoy pushing myself physically and mentally to do what I once thought was not possible. But at some point, I'd expect to embrace a transition to more cerebral activities. I've always enjoyed the mental challenges and sense of fulfillment that writing has provided. It stimulates neuron connections that continue to grow like muscles in my brain. Writing keeps me young by strengthening my mind's neuro pathways. At an earlier time, it was common for me to be in conversation and suddenly draw a blank when trying to remember a name or idea. Those brain farts or senior moments may still occur, but not nearly as often. My ability to recall memories has only gotten better. I've become more aware of the warning signals associated with cognitive issues. Family members will repeat the same stories countless times to the same people without realizing it. The mayoclinic.org website describes dementia as "a group of symptoms affecting memory, thinking and social abilities severely enough to interfere with your daily life." They refer to Alzheimer's disease as "the most common cause of a progressive dementia in older adults." Bartending, personal training, holistic sports nutrition, mortgage loan origination, trading stocks and bonds, Web3 technology, and cryptocurrency were all skills that I had to learn to supplement my income. I may not use them all on a regular basis, but investigating those topics taught me to understand people, global matters, and my place in a rapidly changing world. Learning languages and returning to music are on my current checklist of interests. They provide challenges that will prevent my mind's pathways from becoming rigid in stale thought. Whenever my mind is static for too long, I can feel aging accelerating.

The "golden" years are supposed to be an individual's best productive years after retirement. Sadly, what I see is older people in "developed" countries increasingly struggling to complete simple tasks. Misleading popular catchphrases made more sense after I customized them. I now understand that "health care" is self-accountability for my actions. My decisions have had the greatest impact on my health thus far. No one should be expected to look out for me more than me. I became familiar with my family tree by going back three generations. That was initiated by the habit of getting routine medical checkups. Submitting family medical history was always a requirement during the first meeting with a new doctor. There's valuable information in knowing the dis-eases that past and current family members have suffered from. Doctors only showed interest in my symptoms. I was more intrigued with what caused the symptoms and how to cure them. It took time and effort to pinpoint the causes of those diseases. But it was time well spent. I discovered that genes are not the most important things families share in regard to health. Genes determine where our strengths and weaknesses lie. But the foods we eat and our exercise habits, or lack thereof, actually have a greater influence than our genetic predispositions. For me, the real meaning of modern medicine is eating health-promoting foods indigenous to where my ancestors once thrived. It also requires me to identify foods not compatible with my digestive system. These health-promoting foods promote preventable disease in the family and immediate surroundings. Water-rich foods, on the other hand, are essential, especially in warm, sunny environments. Dis-ease constantly distracts those in their golden years from being able to enjoy the beauty of aging. Miseducation led me to misunderstand the cleverness in nature. The medicine for most of my ailments was in the food all along. Not the foodlike products that tried to imitate nature, but the ones that actually grew out of the soil. It's not by accident that the most nutritious foods come in the most vibrant colors. Once I figured that out, the process of aging became more pleasurable. I took my foot off of the aging accelerator.

I'm no longer obsessed with staying young. Being young has always come naturally to me. I just had to follow my inner voice. I tried to chase the latest trends; it was never fulfilling. As a longtime hip-hop enthusiast and practitioner, I once fell into the quicksand. The commercial dynamic of the middle-aged genre has always promoted younger artists. Males born in my generation started dressing and rapping about things that appealed to younger people. They felt pressure by record labels to appear younger. Many of them had kids the same age as the fan base the record companies were catering to. I was watching and participating in a pre-midlife crisis in real time. I didn't make it this far to be a follower. I have too much life experience during the tough times and the glorious occasions not to let my unique light shine. Engaging in conversation with young people gets me excited. They see the world we live in from a different perspective. The best exchanges happen when we share our distinctive points of view and experiences. Speaking with them about new technology systems is the slang that will influence the way I talk. Not because it sounds good but because it's positively life-changing for global populations.

Fashion comes and goes. Then it comes back around again. So does slang. The new slang words in current pop culture don't flow as freely from me as they do for the generation that uses them daily. I'd sound like a foreigner in my own country. The fabrics and the new fashions don't always fit to my liking. I admired the kids in school who were confident in expressing themselves. Sure, some wore the clothes that the older kids wore first. They shopped at the same stores to get the current brand names. Yes, they were imitating someone else to find an eccentric interpretation of who they really were. Being young at any age is about knowing who you are. It's about knowing who you're not. That becomes clearer when the internal and external toxic energy is removed and kept out of your mind and body. Once the static is gone, it becomes easier to tune in to your distinctive frequency. That vibration connects you to your purpose. That mission is in line with everything else in the universe.

I've never seen cosmetic surgery as an enhancement. I don't know from personal experience, but it sounds like playing a game with no chance of winning. Mother Nature is undefeated and the laws of gravity will always be enforced. If I'm going to put my limited time into activities, it'll be movement. From time to time, I'll watch movies or videos from decades earlier. Fit actors still look attractive and give off great energy no matter what they're wearing. Being fit and healthy doesn't go out of style. We all have an expiration date on this Earth, but certain qualities last much longer than others.

I like my chances of going on aging gracefully if I keep chasing new fitness goals. They're more sustainable than materialistic ones. Financial freedom puts me in a better position to keep my dreams alive. It can also make it easier to help others attain their goals. Making money is essential. Getting lots of money and indulging in gluttony has never seemed appealing to me. The last thing I'd want to do is accelerate aging when money can produce opportunities to gently tap the brakes.

Aging gracefully is being comfortable in my youthful skin. It's about having confidence in the work I've put in over the years and letting that speak. Aging gracefully is standing tall when it comes to my principles and leading by example for future generations. Aging gracefully is saying and expressing everything I have in my heart and backing it up with actions. It's about not having to remember what I said because I'm confident it was what I knew to be the truth.

Staying young has required me to unlearn much of what I was taught and relearn what I already knew. The stimulation I enjoyed after drinking alcohol and smoking drugs was temporary. I continued for years because I was trying to fill voids—the ones created by empty relationships, lack of purpose, low self-esteem, not knowing who I was, and being around people who were trying to figure life out, like I was. A lifestyle that prioritizes movement has always kept me feeling more energized and aging gracefully. Yoga, positive relationships, and enjoying compatible foods have all become nonnegotiable basics. These activities have helped me maintain and build present awareness of a bright future I look forward to.

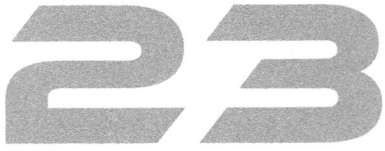

DOWN TO EARTH: MY EARTHING EXPLORATION

To ground is to pour your energies back into the earth and feel the warm calm of nature entering your body in exchange.
— *Anonymous*

I've lived near the Atlantic Ocean for most of my life. Yet I could easily count the number of times I have gone to the beach. I didn't pay much attention to this until I moved down to South Florida. Global lockdown gave me a moment to reflect on the dozens of times I had been in South Beach bars and clubs but never on the sandy side of Ocean Drive. I've always loved to wear sneakers, and that probably won't ever change. But the only times I ever took my shoes off were to shower and sleep. I rarely slept without socks. One weekend, a friend of mine came from out of town to visit and suggested we meet on the beach. Restrictions were gradually being lifted and I was rediscovering the coastline's magnetic attraction. It had been several years, but the sound of waves crashing was so familiar. The madness that was going on around us was eclipsed by the sun, fresh air, and beautiful ocean breeze. It was then that I finally realized I had been missing out on one of nature's greatest tools. Shortly after, I did some reading about earthing, also known as grounding. It's how humans walked the Earth before the normalization of modern footwear. Something as simple as putting bare feet on the Earth's surface improves electrical activity in the brain, enhances blood flow, and counteracts mental illnesses such as anxiety and depression.

I knew that homes and most appliances had to be grounded. But I never really investigated the reasons why. So when I found out that electric current had to flow to the ground to prevent potentially lethal electrical shocks, damage to appliances, and fires, I felt like the only one who didn't know.

Trillions of cells in my body are specialized to conduct electric currents. When the air is dry, they build up static electricity. On occasion I've accidentally shocked a few unsuspecting victims. Electricity flows through my nervous system. Information highways send signals enabling me to think, move, and feel. My body had been on autopilot for so long, I never gave it much thought. I didn't have to. I began to pay closer attention to my surroundings, though. For safety reasons, walking barefoot outdoors these days may require some strategic planning. I made sure to seek surfaces that were regularly exposed to the sun, aka the greatest disinfectant. But even when I was on the beach, many people wore shoes with rubber soles. The problem is, electricity doesn't flow through rubber. It acts as an insulator to keep us from being grounded.

During peak hours at the fitness gym, it was a challenge to find any space to move around. These were the popular times for people to exercise before or after work, and most gravitated toward the treadmills and elliptical machines. They would stare at the screens, moving their feet in a hypnotic rhythm, with people of all ages clutching onto the machine's rails for support due to poor balance and posture. I also noticed that I wasn't the only one who wore shoes way past expiration. It was typical to find shoe soles and heels that were severely worn out. Over time, the uneven distribution of weight and pressure on the feet could cause issues with gait and posture.

This realization helped me understand why hip, back, and neck pain were so common among gym-goers. I, too, was guilty of wearing cushioned shoes for too long, unknowingly encouraging poor walking and running mechanics. Over time, the unused muscles in my feet weakened and lost flexibility. I also observed that some gym members who only came to walk on the machines had the worst postures.

Between seven and ten thousand steps has long been seen as a healthy daily goal for movement. I discovered that walking those steps on the beach barefoot was far more advantageous for me. The wet sand along the coastline not only offered a picturesque view of the ocean but also exposed me to the power of the current. Surfaces like sand, grass, and soil are the liveliest to connect with the Earth's energy field.

Growing up in New York, I developed a fear of stepping on harmful objects like broken glass, cigarette butts, sticky chewing gum, or bodily fluids. Weird, when I think of it. But exposing my bare feet to anything other than the inside of my shoes took some getting used to. On dry sand it was challenging to walk straight while keeping my balance without looking down. The Earth's surfaces were either too hot, too cold, too wet, or just uncomfortable. However, over time, I began to crave the opportunity to remove my shoes and absorb the free ions from the Earth. Although my feet were tender and sensitive at first, I began to feel muscles, tendons, ligaments. and the thousands of nerves under my feet reawaken as I connected with the uneven surface. After a few weeks, I was able to walk and run along the shoreline regularly, feeling more connected with the Earth than ever before.

In general, walking and running have improved my health considerably. But performing these activities barefoot has given me a far better sensory experience. The sights, sounds, smell, and sensations of the ocean are powerful even when the water is calm. Layers of stress melt away from my conscious mind with each step. The Earth naturally balances the electrical functions of all my body's systems. Grounding while moving outdoors is always a refreshing experience.

Water has magnificent memory and can travel great distances. Each time I stood at the edge of the ocean, watching the waves crash against the shore, I couldn't help but wonder if I was reconnecting with water from earlier times in my life. Was I tapping into the memories and experiences that were imprinted onto this very water, long before I even existed? It was a humbling thought—to consider that the very substance that makes up our bodies, the substance that sustains all life on this planet, could hold such incredible power. I couldn't deny the sense of calm and clarity that came with being around it. Maybe I was absorbing information not just from my surroundings in the present moment but from the water itself—from its journey across vast oceans, from the creatures that called it home, from the history that it held within its molecules. And maybe, I was better able to make sense of it now than I ever had been before.

Whether it's neutralizing free radicals that influence inflammation, combating insomnia, high blood pressure, stress, or other imbalances, grounding is another simple yet underrated course of action to not accelerate the inevitable process of aging. It's become a lost art, like other things I did when I was younger. Whenever I'm within reasonable distance, time on the beach has become a priority for me.

> **GEMS:** As great as it could be to walk around with bare feet all day, it may not be practical in most urban settings. I set aside time whenever possible to connect my soles with the Earth's soul. I've also noticed that as the miles I run in shoes have increased, my foot pain, blisters, and even injuries have gone down. The uneven distribution of weight and pressure on my feet used to cause issues with gait and posture. Grounding has helped to reverse these problems.

24
FINAL THOUGHTS

Education is the most powerful weapon which you can use to change the world.
— *Nelson Mandela*

As I look back on my life, I realize that the pursuit of youth has always been something I valued. Not just physical youth but the youthful spirit that allows us to see the world with wonder and amazement. It's a quality that I've always admired in others and longed for in myself. And as I've grown older, I've come to realize that staying young is not just about vanity or superficial concerns; it's a way of showing gratitude and valuing the world around us.

One of the most important things I've learned on my journey is that the health of the Earth and its diverse life-forms are intimately connected with our well-being. It's easy to get caught up in the hustle and bustle of everyday life and forget about the bigger picture, but I've come to understand that we need to take a holistic approach to our health if we want to truly prevent premature aging.

Scientists will continue to search for various ways to manipulate genes and regenerate our telomeres, the tips at the ends of our DNA. These telomeres keep our DNA from unraveling like the plastic tips on the end of a shoe's laces. Telomere length tends to shorten as we age, which is a natural part of the aging process that begins from the moment we're born. I've seen firsthand how some people are willing to gamble on quick fixes and fad diets, only to end up disappointed when they realize that these short-term solutions don't last. Aging brings natural challenges no one can evade. Still, I believe we each have unique gifts to meet those challenges and express ourselves.

Unfortunately, society as a whole is aging prematurely due to self-inflicted habits. But there are proven methods that can help us age more gracefully. For me, this has meant seeking out the advice of doctors and remaining consistent in my fitness routine. I've had my ups and downs over the years, but I've never gone more than a few months without some form of resistance training. It's not always easy, but the results are worth it. Our bodies are designed to repair and grow stronger, and I've seen the benefits of pushing myself to my limits.

But fitness is just one piece of the puzzle. Clean water is another crucial component of good health, and it's something that is becoming increasingly difficult to find. With pollution from fossil fuels, pesticides, and man-made chemicals, it's more important than ever to seek out fresh, organic fruits and vegetables that can act as natural filters. And while it's true that animal agriculture uses up a significant portion of our water supply, we can all do our part to reduce our impact and find sustainable solutions.

Fresh air is also essential for good health. The benefits of consistently making time to breathe deeply outdoors is underrated. Diverse microorganisms that are only found outdoors can enhance the body's resilience against disease. As I writer I'm well aware of the temptation to sit in chairs for extended periods of time. Breathing outdoor air every day is essential for me to maintain my cognitive function and overall productivity. With air pollution on the rise, it's becoming increasingly important to take action to reduce our carbon footprint and protect our planet. And as we saw with the lockdown events in 2020, even small changes in our habits make a big difference in carbon dioxide emissions. Sometimes I wonder if I'll have to purchase clean air to breathe someday. When I was a kid, I'd regularly ride to the gas station to fill my basketballs, footballs, and bicycle tires with air. Many places now charge a fee. I never imagined that I'd have to pay for air. I've been able to find some alternatives online. Freeairpump.com provides a user-generated database of the few places going against the trend.

Life purpose is a journey that has brought me immense joy and fulfillment by sharing beneficial information through writing. At times, I doubted if it was too late for me to make an impact, but life has taught me that it's never too late to pursue your passion. The satisfaction of completing a passionate project further fuels my desire to achieve more and set new goals for myself.

I may not live long enough to see a world where everyone follows the steps outlined in this book, but it is my hope that in the future people will endeavor to adopt a healthier diet and lifestyle. Real progress will require the most powerful nations to take the lead, but unfortunately, they are causing the most environmental damage, limiting the options for future generations. However, I believe humanity can unite and learn from those on the successful path to create a better world.

This book represents a culmination of experiences that have shaped my being, instilling within me a fervent desire to draw attention to the preventable diseases that afflict so many. The words within these pages hold the potential to bestow meaningful benefits upon those who are receptive to them. Although my story is unique, the symptoms I have endured are tragically all too prevalent in our world.

Information that was once easy to find on search engines and media platforms are now being censored by corporations with strategic partnerships. It's more important than ever for individuals to study their environment and learn as much as possible.

Humans have not changed much anatomically since the earliest *Homo sapiens* roamed the Earth, and scientists have proved that they thrived on a plant-dominant diet. However, global conditions have dramatically changed, and humans continuously experiment with food substances that are not compatible with our anatomy, resulting in a diet that makes disease inevitable. More of the food supply is being controlled by individuals with selfish agendas. The urgency for the majority to support local farmers and grow their own produce has never been higher.

The sun is the source of life on this planet, and my life improved once I began to view exposure to sunlight as important as any other vital nutrient. My ancestors came from near the equator, and the sun will always play a prominent role in wellness.

I am not a medical professional, but I would advise all those who are concerned about their health to research for themselves and communicate with qualified health-care professionals. Almost anyone can be young at any age as long as that person desires good health and keeps an open mind.

Many of us endure long-term pain in attempts to chase short-term gain, but there are no shortcuts to great health. Numerous steps are necessary to prevent premature aging, including growing your own food, meditation, and physically pushing the body consistently while having fun. We're not perfect beings. Being able to juggle many things all of the time is just not realistic for most of us. The goal for me is to learn more, apply more, and get better. If I can do that and share knowledge that can help someone else, then life has more purpose.

Working with a holistic, lifestyle-centered physician can help identify the location and stage of any symptoms you may encounter. Once I understood the strengths and limitations of traditional medical doctors, I became much more confident in my ability to overcome common issues. By doing my own research. I was able to have more intelligent, advantageous conversations with medical professionals. I was able to help them to assist me in finding the causes and cures of these issues.

A fulfilling life springs from simple pleasures and good health. When we nourish our bodies with wholesome foods, pursue meaningful goals with passion, enjoy the warmth of the sun, sleep well, drink pure water, breathe the freshest air available, move our bodies, and have fun, we thrive. Those around us may take note of our vitality, though some may not understand our choices. That's okay - we each walk our own path in this life. While our beliefs differ, kindness and respect for one another remain paramount. When our time comes, we all return to the earth. Until then, may we celebrate the diversity that makes us human.

There are no secrets to being young at any age, and no amount of money put into antiaging wonder drugs will safely prolong someone's life span. However, there's information that many of us haven't been exposed to previously, and younger generations need exposure to nutritional science during their grade-school years. This may require like-minded individuals to form communities that build places of learning to teach these and other fundamental life skills. Becoming one with our environment and discovering our individual and collective roles to preserve this planet is key. The importance of returning to natural living to reconnect and disconnect from stressful, useless material possessions cannot be overstated.

Finally, rest and sleep are just as important as exercise and nutrition when it comes to aging gracefully. For years, I used to believe that sleep was a waste of time, but I've come to understand that it's an essential part of the recharging process. Without adequate sleep, I can't be the best version of myself, and I've made plenty of poor decisions in the past as a result.

The pursuit of youth is a pursuit of self-worth. It is a commitment to cherishing our bodies, our loved ones, and the fleeting gift of time. Though we cannot halt the steady march of age, we can refuse to accelerate our decline. The path ahead holds both sorrow and joy. With wisdom, we may avoid preventable pains and savor life's sweetness. My humble wish is to have shared some lasting GEMS that light your way. For the measure of our days is not their quantity, but the quality we instill in them. Embrace this moment. The world is ours.

SOURCES

https://www.mayoclinic.org/diseases-conditions/progeria/symptoms-causes/syc-20356038

https://www.latimes.com/opinion/op-ed/la-oe-reiss-race-sleep-gap-20170423-story.html

https://www.nejm.org/doi/pdf/10.1056/NEJMoa1306357

https://www.cell.com/ajhg/fulltext/S0002-9297(18)30363-X

https://www.sciencedaily.com/releases/2012/06/120627131931.htm

https://www.slavevoyages.org/tast/index.faces

https://www.cdc.gov/pcd/issues/2017/17_0153.htm

https://www.theguardian.com/environment/2020/mar/23/coronavirus-pandemic-leading-to-huge-drop-in-air-pollution

https://www.ncbi.nlm.nih.gov/pmc/articles/PMC5613902/

https://pubmed.ncbi.nlm.nih.gov/20522508/

https://pubmed.ncbi.nlm.nih.gov/12528966/

https://www.ncbi.nlm.nih.gov/pmc/articles/PMC3650511/

https://www.ncbi.nlm.nih.gov/pmc/articles/PMC4784299/

https://diabetesjournals.org/care/article/41/8/1732/36380/Saturated-Fat-Is-More-Metabolically-Harmful-for

https://data.worldbank.org/indicator/SP.DYN.LE00.MA.IN?end=2020&locations=HT&start=1970

https://nutritionfacts.org/video/sodium-and-arterial-function-a-salting-our-endothelium/

EXERCISES TO IMPROVE POSTURE

You are advised to consult your physician before making any dietary changes. Before beginning any new exercise program, consult a health professional. Stop immediately if you experience pain.

Have you ever noticed an elderly stranger on the street or in a car and instinctively known their age from their stooped posture? Or conversely, assumed someone was younger than their years because they stood tall? Rounded thoracic spine; poor posture due to staring at portable devices or sitting for too long is a growing trend. Below are some basic movements to help improve posture.

Wall slides - Stand with your back against a wall, feet hip-width apart. Keep your back, head, and arms against the wall while sliding your arms up overhead. Then, bend your elbows to 90 degrees and slide them back down. Repeat for a few reps to improve shoulder mobility and posture.

Face pulls w/ TRX or rope - Stand facing the anchor point holding a TRX or rope with an overhand grip. Step back to create tension, feet shoulder-width apart. Pull the handles toward your face, squeezing shoulder blades together. Keep core engaged, elbows out. Return to starting position with control. Repeat for desired reps.

Shoulder Circles - To perform bodyweight shoulder circles, stand with feet shoulder-width apart, raise both arms out to the sides, and make small circular motions with your shoulders. Keep the movements controlled and repeat in both clockwise and counterclockwise directions. Avoid arching your back and engage your core throughout.

Shoulder Shrugs - Stand with feet shoulder-width apart, arms down by your sides. Elevate shoulders towards ears, hold for a moment, then lower them back down. Keep a neutral spine and avoid using momentum. Repeat for desired reps to strengthen the trapezius muscles. For more resistance, hold a weight in each hand.

Floor Planks - Assume a plank position on the floor with forearms and toes supporting the body. Keep a straight line from head to heels, engage core muscles, and hold for a set duration while maintaining proper form and breathing.

RECIPES

Included here are some of my favorite things to eat.

BANANA/BLUEBERRY NICE CREAM

Ingredients

- Ripe bananas
- Fresh or frozen blueberries
- Coconut water or spring water

Preparation

Allow bananas to ripen fully. You will know when they are soft to the touch and covered with brown/black spots. These spots indicate increased sweetness, antioxidants, and digestibility. Unpeel bananas, break apart into two-inch pieces, place in a bag, and put into a freezer until frozen.

Remove bananas from freezer and place as many as you like into a blender, with as many blueberries as you like. Fill blender container up halfway with coconut water or spring water and blend for up to a minute. The final consistency should resemble a smooth shake, requiring the use of a spoon to eat. Enjoy!

A University of California, Davis study researched how blending smoothie ingredients affects flavonoid absorption. Although banana-berry smoothies decreased flavonoid levels in the participants, I've had success with banana-blueberry smoothies and enjoy the taste.

MINT CHOCOLATE CHIP NICE CREAM

Ingredients

- 1–2 tablespoons of fresh mint leaves
- Frozen bananas
- 2 tablespoons of raw cacao nibs
- Coconut water or spring water

Preparation

Place as many frozen bananas as you like into a blender, with two tablespoons of raw cacao nibs and fresh mint leaves. Fill blender container up halfway with coconut water or spring water and blend for up to a minute. The final consistency should resemble a smooth shake, requiring the use of a spoon to eat. Enjoy!

GOOD GREEN SMOOTHIE

Ingredients

- 1–2 Medjool dates
- 1 or 2 ripe, frozen bananas (break into smaller pieces before placing in containers and freezing.)
- A 50/50% mixture of de-stemmed kale and spinach leaves (I usually fill the craft halfway to the top with greens.)
- Coconut water or unsweetened non-dairy milk (I usually pour up to the level of the greens...about halfway to the top.)
- 1 small thin slice of fresh ginger or turmeric
- 1 teaspoon of vanilla extract

Preparation

Fill blender craft halfway to the top with the mixture of greens. Add frozen bananas into a blender, with the slice of fresh ginger or turmeric and dates. Fill blender container up halfway with coconut water or non-dairy milk and blend on high until smooth. The final consistency should resemble a smooth shake, requiring the use of a spoon to eat. Enjoy!

BLACK BEAN BURGER

Ingredients

- 2 cups cooked black beans, drained and rinsed
- ½ cup cooked quinoa
- ¼ cup diced cilantro
- ½ cup diced red onion
- 2 tbsp tomato paste
- 2 cloves minced garlic
- 2 tbsp ground cumin
- 2 tbsp nutritional yeast
- 1 tbsp smoked paprika
- 1 tbsp onion powder

Preparation

Preheat oven to 375°F.
Mash black beans in a mixing bowl with a fork until they form a chunky mush.
Add the rest of the ingredients and mix together thoroughly.
Form 4–6 burger patties.
Place patties on a baking sheet lined with parchment paper. Bake for 25–30 minutes. Flip once after 15 minutes.
Top with your choice of kale, lettuce, tomato, pickles, avocado, etc.

Serve with a salad or on Ezekiel sprouted bread.

JUST LIKE SOY SAUCE

Ingredients

- 1 large celery stalk
- 1 large tomato
- 1 oz of shelled and seeded sweet tamarind
- A squeeze of lime

Preparation

Blend all ingredients together.

This recipe is a great way to get the soy sauce flavor without the high amounts of salt.

BASIL PESTO

Ingredients

- 3 cloves of garlic
- 1½ cup of green peas
- 1 medium red onion or 3 green onions
- ½ cup of basil
- 2 cups of spinach
- ½ cup of lime or lemon juice

Preparation

Blend ingredients and pour over zucchini noodles.
Garnish with bell peppers and 1 diced Hass avocado

RED TOMATO DRESSING

Ingredients

- 1 large tomato
- 3 dates
- 2 green onions
- 2 stalks of celery
- 6 sun-dried tomatoes
- half an avocado
- 5 basil leaves

Preparation

Blend all ingredients together to pour over a green salad.

HUMMUS

Ingredients

- 3 cups of garbanzo beans soaked in water for 8 hours
- 1 cup of sesame seeds
- 1 1/2 cups of lemon juice
- 3 cloves of garlic
- 1 cup of water

Preparation

Blend ingredients together to eat with celery, carrots, etc. Sprinkle paprika on top.

RANCH DRESSING

Ingredients

- 1 1/2 cups of hemp seeds
- 1 cup of water
- 1 tsp of nutritional yeast
- 1 tsp of powdered onion
- 2 tsp of powdered garlic
- 4 tbsp of lemon juice
- 1 tsp of apple cider vinegar
- Optional: Add parsley and dill.

Preparation

Blend ingredients together to consistency of your liking.

VEGETABLE SALADS

A large vegetable salad at the end of the day has been working well for me. The ingredients vary according to the season. I also like to rotate the greens I'm eating to make sure I'm consuming different ratios of nutrients. Kale, collard greens, watercress, bok choy, spinach, katuk, and romaine lettuce are some of my favorite green leafy vegetables. I let my body's systems take care of the nutrient distribution. All ingredients are soaked in baking soda for 5-10 minutes to remove the surface-level chemicals, rinsed and diced up into a bowl. The amount of salad varies according to my activity level during the day. Multiply ingredients for each additional person.

Ingredients

- 1 head of Romaine Lettuce
- 1 Red Bell Pepper
- 1 stalk of Celery

- 1 Cucumber
- 1 bunch of Watercress
- 1 Tomato
- 1 Carrot
- Garbanzo Beans (1-2 cans- No Sodium Added)
- Hass Avocado. (Lemon for dressing)

BLOOMED WILD RICE

Score as much wild rice as you like for 1 minute in a food processor until the wild rice is completely covered with black powder, no pulsing. The process of scoring cuts the hard surface of the hard rice to allow it to soak up more water and soften more quickly.

Next, rinse the wild rice thoroughly under water until the water turns clear. Place wild rice into a half gallon–size mason jar.

Pour in water and let soak for 12–18 hours.

Ensure that the jar has enough room for the wild rice to expand 3 or 4 times. 16 oz of wild rice can fill up a half-gallon jar in 18 hours.

Drain and rinse well.

The wild rice can be seasoned with your favorite herbs, gently steamed with broccoli, mushrooms or paired with beans.

SIMPLE QUIZ QUESTIONS

1. How much water should men and women drink daily?

    A. 5 cups/3 cups
    B. 6 cups/4 cups
    C. 13 cups/9 cups
    D. 20 cups/18 cups

2. What foods can help to alleviate insulin resistance?

    A. Kale
    B. Arugula
    C. Watercress
    D. All of the above

3. What are some potential benefits of a juice or water fast?

    A. The digestive organs in the body are given time to rest.
    B. Eliminating toxins becomes the main focus of the body.
    C. Fruit juices can help cleanse and energize the body.
    D. All of the above

4. What activities can be good for helping to relieve stress?

    A. Getting involved with social activities
    B. Avoiding caffeine and alcohol
    C. Getting a massage
    D. All of the above

5. What is necessary for success on a lifestyle change journey?

    A. Inspiration

B. Motivation
C. Knowing what to do and how to do it
D. Discipline
E. All of the above.

ANSWERS

1. C: The National Academy of Medicine recommends 13 cups for healthy men and 9 cups for healthy women.
2. D: All of the above.
3. D: All of the above.
4. D: All of the above.
5. E: All of the above.

ACKNOWLEDGEMENTS

Beta Readers – Terrance Ferguson, Sara Pierce, Anderson Vilien, Laurie Stark, Michael Stoute, Rodney Jean Bart, and Charles Loiseau. Thank you for reading my early drafts when I was still struggling to shape my words on the page. Your insightful questions and suggestions helped me to find focus when the writing felt distorted.

Audience – Monday's memoir writing workshop in the Bienes Museum Conference Room was being at the right place in the right time. Some of the best listeners and talented writers I've ever met. Authentic feedback from attentive, undistracted people with international experience can be challenging to locate but is what every writer needs. Retrieving memories and putting them into words became a fun challenge every month.

Kevin Powell – Your words of encouragement and willingness to share suggestions and resources assisted in my evolution as a writer. The weekly writing workshops reignited my passion for writing at a time when my dedication to the craft was dim and needed a jumpstart.

Rose Nesmy Saint-Louis– Our conversations about the limitless forms of artistic expression, trusting the natural process of creation, and the commitment to staying on the path to fulfill our mission have been truly priceless.

Drew Spence – Thank you for decades of stalwart friendship.

Special thank you to Steve Vaccaro, Jill Martin and the entire Chapters Network team.

WILL LOISEAU

To my readers, who have embraced my style and subject matters. Your unshakable backing and support continue to fuel my creative spirit. This book is dedicated to every one of you.

ABOUT THE AUTHOR

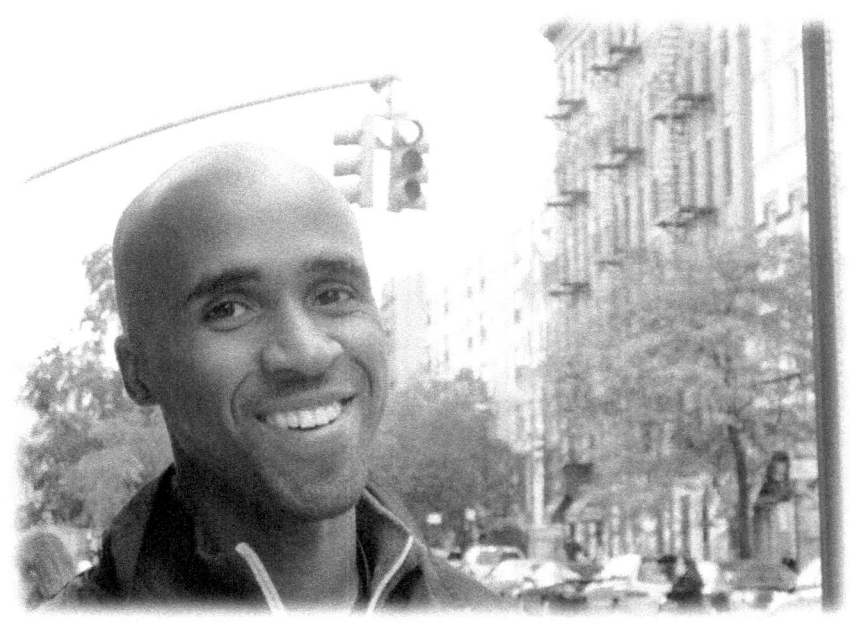

Photo Credit: Jonathan Mok.

Brooklyn-born writer Will Loiseau found his calling amidst calamity. Though his innate gift for storytelling emerged in childhood, he initially pursued a scientific path, studying to become a physical therapist. But the seeds of his literary future took root when a college English professor recognized his talent.

Years later, while processing a traumatic experience abroad through writing, Will uncovered his authentic voice. Turning disaster into prose, he published

WILL LOISEAU

"QUAKE"--a gripping firsthand account of surviving the devastating 2010 Haitian earthquake.

When he isn't writing, Will is an avid runner and certified sports nutritionist motivating others toward healthy lifestyles. He captivates readers with his unique background, overcoming adversity through resilience. With lyrical prose and an inspiring true story, Will Loiseau is making waves in the literary scene.

Thank you for reading. If you found this book to be of any value, I would be grateful if you could spread the good word and refer it to someone who could appreciate it.

Best of health,

Will

TrueIronWill.com

www.ingramcontent.com/pod-product-compliance
Lightning Source LLC
Chambersburg PA
CBHW060946050426
42337CB00052B/1616